*Etzel Cardeña, PhD*
*Kristin Croyle, PhD*
*Editors*

# Acute Reactions to Trauma and Psychotherapy: A Multidisciplinary and International Perspective

*Acute Reactions to Trauma and Psychotherapy: A Multidisciplinary and International Perspective* has been co-published simultaneously as *Journal of Trauma & Dissociation*, Volume 6, Number 2 2005.

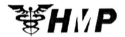

The Haworth Medical Press®
An Imprint of The Haworth Press, Inc.

# Acute Reactions to Trauma and Psychotherapy: A Multidisciplinary and International Perspective

*Acute Reactions to Trauma and Psychotherapy: A Multidisciplinary and International Perspective* has been co-published simultaneously as *Journal of Trauma & Dissociation*, Volume 6, Number 2 2005.

## Monographic Separates from the *Journal of Trauma & Dissociation*

For additional information on these and other Haworth Press titles, including descriptions, tables of contents, reviews, and prices, use the QuickSearch catalog at http://www.HaworthPress.com.

*Acute Reactions to Trauma and Psychotherapy: A Multidisciplinary and International Perspective,* edited by Etzel Cardeña, PhD, and Kristin Croyle, PhD (Vol. 6, No. 2, 2005). *"COMPREHENSIVE, INFORMATIVE.... CONCISE AND WELL WRITTEN.... A wonderful introduction to a summary of current knowledge about acute stress reactions.... A USEFUL RESOURCE FOR GRADUATE STUDENTS as well as for trauma and other mental health researchers and practitioners.... Covers a wide range of relevant issues, including vulnerabilities and risk factors, diagnosis, effects of acute stress reactions on the brain, treatment, the role of coping, and peritraumatic dissociation. The research reported here crosses a range of potentially traumatic events and experiences such as house fires, terrorist attacks, and burns." (Laurie Anne Pearlman, PhD, Co-Director, Traumatic Stress Institute/Center for Adult & Adolescent Psychotherapy LLC)*

*Trauma and Sexuality: The Effects of Childhood Sexual, Physical, and Emotional Abuse on Sexual Identity and Behavior,* edited by James A. Chu, MD, and Elizabeth S. Bowman, MD (Vol. 3, No. 4, 2002). *Examines the effects of childhood trauma on sexual orientation and behavior.*

# Acute Reactions to Trauma and Psychotherapy: A Multidisciplinary and International Perspective

Etzel Cardeña, PhD
Kristin Croyle, PhD
Editors

*Acute Reactions to Trauma and Psychotherapy: A Multidisciplinary and International Perspective* has been co-published simultaneously as *Journal of Trauma & Dissociation*, Volume 6, Number 2 2005.

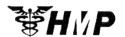

The Haworth Medical Press®
The Haworth Maltreatment & Trauma Press®
Imprints of The Haworth Press, Inc.

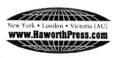

New York • London • Victoria (AU)
www.HaworthPress.com

Published by

The Haworth Medical Press®, 10 Alice Street, Binghamton, NY 13904-1580 USA

The Haworth Medical Press® is an imprint of The Haworth Press, Inc., 10 Alice Street, Binghamton, NY 13904-1580 USA.

*Acute Reactions to Trauma and Psychotherapy: A Multidisciplinary and International Perspective* has been co-published simultaneously as *Journal of Trauma & Dissociation*, Volume 6, Number 2 2005.

The development, preparation, and publication of this work has been undertaken with great care. However, the publisher, employees, editors, and agents of The Haworth Press and all imprints of The Haworth Press, Inc., including The Haworth Medical Press® and Pharmaceutical Products Press®, are not responsible for any errors contained herein or for consequences that may ensue from use of materials or information contained in this work. Opinions expressed by the author(s) are not necessarily those of The Haworth Press, Inc. With regard to case studies, identities and circumstances of individuals discussed herein have been changed to protect confidentiality. Any resemblance to actual persons, living or dead, is entirely coincidental.

Cover design by Lora Wiggins.

**Library of Congress Cataloging-in-Publication Data**

Acute reactions to trauma and psychotherapy : a multidisciplinary and international perspective / Etzel Cardeña, Kristin Croyle, editors.
     p. cm. – (Journal of trauma & dissociation ; v. 6, no. 2)
    Includes bibliographical references and index.
    ISBN-13: 978-0-7890-2973-7 (hard : alk. paper)
    ISBN-10: 0-7890-2973-1 (hard : alk. paper)
    ISBN-13: 978-0-7890-2974-4 (pbk. : alk.paper)
    ISBN-10: 0-7890-2974-X (pbk. : alk.paper)
    1. Stress (Psychology) 2. Post-traumatic stress disorder.
    I. Cardeña, Etzel. II. Croyle, Kristin. III. Series.
[DNLM: 1. Stress Disorders, Post-Traumatic. 2. Terrorism–psychology. WM 170 A189 2005]
RC455.4.S87A25 2005
629.44'2–dc22
                                              2005001491

# Indexing, Abstracting & Website/Internet Coverage

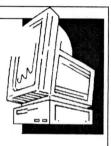

    This section provides you with a list of major indexing & abstracting services and other tools for bibliographic access. That is to say, each service began covering this periodical during the year noted in the right column. Most Websites which are listed below have indicated that they will either post, disseminate, compile, archive, cite or alert their own Website users with research-based content from this work. (This list is as current as the copyright date of this publication.)

Abstracting, Website/Indexing Coverage . . . . . . . . Year When Coverage Began

- *Biology Digest (in print & online) <http://www.infotoday.com>* . . **2000**
- *Business Source Corporate: coverage of nearly 3,350 quality magazines and journals; designed to meet the diverse information needs of corporations; EBSCO Publishing <http://www.epnet.com/corporate/bsourcecorp.asp>* . . . . . . . . **2003**
- *Contemporary Women's Issues* . . . . . . . . . . . . . . . . . . . . . . . . . . **2000**
- *EAP Abstracts Plus <http://www.eaptechnology.com>* . . . . . . . . . **2000**
- *EBSCOhost Electronic Journals Service (EJS) <http://ejournals.ebsco.com>* . . . . . . . . . . . . . . . . . . . . . . . . . . . **2001**
- *EMBASE.com (The Power of EMBASE + MEDLINE Combined) <http://www.embase.com>* . . . . . . . . . . . . . . . . . . . . . . . . . . . . **2000**
- *EMBASE/Excerpta Medica Secondary Publishing Division <http://www.elsevier.nl>* . . . . . . . . . . . . . . . . . . . . . . . . . . . . . . **2000**
- *Excerpta Medica . . . See EMBASE* . . . . . . . . . . . . . . . . . . . . . . **2000**
- *e-psyche, LLC <http://www.e-psyche.net>* . . . . . . . . . . . . . . . . . **2001**
- *Family & Society Studies Worldwide <http://www.nisc.com>* . . . . **2000**
- *Google <http://www.google.com>* . . . . . . . . . . . . . . . . . . . . . . . . **2004**
- *Google Scholar <http://scholar.google.com>* . . . . . . . . . . . . . . . **2004**

(continued)

(continued)

*Special Bibliographic Notes related to special journal issues (separates) and indexing/abstracting:*

- indexing/abstracting services in this list will also cover material in any "separate" that is co-published simultaneously with Haworth's special thematic journal issue or DocuSerial. Indexing/abstracting usually covers material at the article/chapter level.
- monographic co-editions are intended for either non-subscribers or libraries which intend to purchase a second copy for their circulating collections.
- monographic co-editions are reported to all jobbers/wholesalers/approval plans. The source journal is listed as the "series" to assist the prevention of duplicate purchasing in the same manner utilized for books-in-series.
- to facilitate user/access services all indexing/abstracting services are encouraged to utilize the co-indexing entry note indicated at the bottom of the first page of each article/chapter/contribution.
- this is intended to assist a library user of any reference tool (whether print, electronic, online, or CD-ROM) to locate the monographic version if the library has purchased this version but not a subscription to the source journal.
- individual articles/chapters in any Haworth publication are also available through the Haworth Document Delivery Service (HDDS).

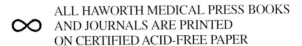

# Acute Reactions to Trauma and Psychotherapy: A Multidisciplinary and International Perspective

## CONTENTS

# ABOUT THE EDITORS

**Etzel Cardeña, PhD,** is Thorsen Chair of Psychology at the University of Lund, Sweden. He got his PhD at the University of California, Davis, and was postdoctoral fellow at Stanford University. He is past chair of his department and past-president of both the Society for Clinical and Experimental Hypnosis and Division 30 of the American Psychological Association. His empirical and theoretical work on acute reactions to trauma and hypnosis has garnered awards from those organizations and from the International Society for the Study of Dissociation and the University of Texas-Pan American. Along with David Spiegel, MD, he proposed in 1991 a diagnosis for acute reactions to trauma, which was introduced into the DSM-IV as Acute Stress Disorder. He also co-authored a widely used instrument for acute reactions to trauma, the Stanford Acute Stress Reaction Questionnaire. He has more than 100 publications, some of them in the top journals of psychology, psychiatry and traumatology. He has also edited two books with the American Psychological Association, *Clinical Hypnosis and Self Regulation*, and *Varieties of Anomalous Experience* ("This is an extraordinary volume, head and shoulders above anything previously written on the topic." Robert Morris, Koestler Chair, University of Edinburgh).

**Kristin Croyle, PhD,** is an Assistant Professor fo Psychology at the University of Texas-Pan American in Edinburg, Texas. She received her PhD in clinical psychology from the University of Montana (2000), following which she completed a postdoctoral residency in clinical neuropsychology at the University of Washington School of Medicine. Her research focuses on the influence of neuropsychological dysfunction on coping with chronic illness, and self-harm in nonclinical populations.

# Introduction:
# Early Trauma Responses and Psychopathology: Setting Up the Stage

Research on short- and long-term response to trauma has been expanding over the past twenty years and has found new urgency in recent national and international events. As our understanding of risk factors for who will be most severely affected by trauma expands, what we *don't* know about the interactions between vulnerabilities and risk factors, peritraumatic and posttraumatic factors, physiological and psychological factors becomes more apparent. An international consensus conference on "Early Trauma Responses and Psychopathology: Theoretical and Empirical Directions," co-sponsored by the National Institute of Mental Health (NIMH), the University of Texas-Pan American, and the National Center for Posttraumatic Stress Disorder (NCPTSD) was planned for September 24-25, 2001. The events of 9/11/2001 tragically showed the relevance of the conference, and forced its rescheduling for 2002. The event had the participation of eminent contributors from Australia, Israel, the United Kingdom, and the United States. This volume anthologizes many of these original contributions.

The workshop organizers–Etzel Cardeña, PhD, Regina Dolan-Sewell, PhD, Terry Keane, PhD, Farris Tuma, PhD, and Robert Ursano, MD–set a conference agenda that included the following issues: terminology and definitions, diagnostic issues, evaluation of acute psychological and biological reactions to trauma, risk factors for acute and chronic psychopathology, and prevention and early intervention. With respect to diagnostic issues and evaluation, various participants agreed that the

[Haworth co-indexing entry note]: "Introduction: Early Trauma Responses and Psychopathology: Setting Up the Stage." Cardeña, Etzel, and Kristin Croyle. Co-published simultaneously in *Journal of Trauma & Dissociation* (The Haworth Medical Press, an imprint of The Haworth Press, Inc.) Vol. 6, No. 2, 2005, pp. 1-3; and: *Acute Reactions to Trauma and Psychotherapy: A Multidisciplinary and International Perspective* (ed: Etzel Cardeña, and Kristin Croyle) The Haworth Medical Press, an imprint of The Haworth Press, Inc., 2005, pp. 1-3. Single or multiple copies of this article are available for a fee from The Haworth Document Delivery Service [1-800-HAWORTH, 9:00 a.m. - 5:00 p.m. (EST). E-mail address: docdelivery@haworthpress.com].

Available online at http://www.haworthpress.com/web/JTD
doi:10.1300/J229v06n02_01

type of trauma (e.g., natural disaster versus, child abuse victims) has a defining impact on acute reactions, and that future research should include prospective, longitudinal, and large sample studies, where functional impairment, biological abnormalities, and medical factors are evaluated along with symptomatology. Participants mentioned the following topics as deserving additional attention and appropriate funding: research with children and juveniles, risk factors and variables predicting resiliency, brain plasticity and gene expression during the first few weeks after exposure to trauma, and the comparison of current and alternative Acute Stress Disorder (ASD) and Posttraumatic Stress Disorder (PTSD) symptom clusters. Recommendations for intervention and treatment included developing effective prevention strategies and evaluating specific therapeutic elements (e.g., cognitive restructuring and other techniques, patient and therapist variables) for their effectiveness or possible iatrogenic effects. Many contributors also remarked on the problem with current funding practices, which make it very difficult to support research of acute reactions to unexpected, traumatic events.

The papers in this volume provide an excellent overview of the state of the literature on acute reactions to trauma. They provide an integrative summary of factors listed above, and provide immediately useful recommendations for further research and clinical interventions among both children and adults.

## DIAGNOSIS AND EVALUATION

Richard Bryant's paper on the relationship between acute reactions and later PTSD opens the issue with a focus on the immediate aftermath of trauma. He provides a clear, succinct summary of ASD, including its utility and limitations. Betty Pfefferbaum provides an insightful discussion of the stressor criterion, necessary for diagnoses of both PTSD and ASD, whereas Carol North describes critical issues in longitudinal disaster research, illustrating her points with data from survivors of the Oklahoma City bombing (April 19, 1995). Glenn Saxe and colleagues describe their findings regarding risk factors for ASD in children with burns. Their project is a strong and well-designed addition to the under-researched area of acute stress reactions in children, and integrates both physiological and behavioral/psychological factors. Douglas Bremner completes this section with a discussion of the relationship between traumatic history and brain structure and function. He includes an interesting recommendation that susceptible brain areas may provide an area of intervention in the immediate aftermath of trauma.

## RISK AND PROCESS FACTORS

Etzel Cardeña and collaborators provide data on acute stress reactions to 9/11 in juveniles and adults from a large, nationwide representative sample. The results highlight the greater importance of coping factors and TV watching over demographic variables. Russell Jones and his co-author focus on children and adolescents' adjustment following residential fire with a particular emphasis on avoidant coping. Their suggestions for organizing risk factors both conceptually and temporally, and for distinguishing risk factors from vulnerability factors provide guidance to further work in this area.

## PREVENTION AND EARLY INTERVENTION

Bridging research and intervention recommendations, David Spiegel summarizes various dimensions of acute stress reactions, course of symptom recovery, components of interventions, and outcome assessment, calling for a more integrative and broader take on outcome research. Judy Cohen contributes to this broader approach with her summary of the treatment of traumatized children, with specific recommendations for clinical practice, research, and public policy in the area. Chris Brewin concludes the special issue with a paper that discusses findings regarding the usefulness of pre-trauma factors and subjective accounts of the severity of the trauma for predicting later PTSD. He concludes with recommendations for a "Screen and Treat" approach that is fully described in his article.

Together these papers form an impressive collection whose main purpose is to stimulate and direct further research. But their applicability does not end there. They also provide succinct and usable clinical recommendations, demonstrating the authors' awareness that those who are traumatized cannot wait for further research.

*Etzel Cardeña, PhD*
*Thorsen Chair of Psychology*
*University of Lund*
*Lund, Sweden*

*Kristin Croyle, PhD*
*Department of Psychology and Anthropology*
*University of Texas-Pan American*
*Edinburg, TX 78539-2999*

# Predicting Posttraumatic Stress Disorder from Acute Reactions

Richard A. Bryant, PhD

**SUMMARY.** There is much interest in identifying people shortly after trauma exposure who will subsequently develop posttraumatic stress disorder (PTSD). This review outlines recent developments in early identification of trauma-exposed people who are at high risk for PTSD development, including the rationale, evidence, and limitations of the acute stress diagnosis as a predictor of chronic PTSD. The potential role of acute dissociative responses mediating development of PTSD is also reviewed. The available evidence suggests that whereas acute dissociation is an important factor in the acute stress response, many people develop PTSD in the absence of dissociative symptoms. The evidence suggests that dissociation needs to be considered in the context of other factors in the aftermath of trauma if optimal identification of high-risk individuals is to be achieved. *[Article copies available for a fee from The Haworth Document Delivery Service: 1-800-HAWORTH. E-mail address: <docdelivery@haworthpress.com> Website: <http://www.HaworthPress.com> © 2005 by The Haworth Press, Inc. All rights reserved.]*

**KEYWORDS.** Acute stress disorder, dissociation, PTSD

Richard A. Bryant is affiliated with the University of New South Wales, Sydney, NSW, Australia.

Address correspondence to: Richard A. Bryant, PhD, School of Psychology, University of New South Wales, NSW, 2052, Australia (E-mail: r.bryant@unsw.edu.au).

[Haworth co-indexing entry note]: "Predicting Posttraumatic Stress Disorder from Acute Reactions." Bryant, Richard A. Co-published simultaneously in *Journal of Trauma & Dissociation* (The Haworth Medical Press, an imprint of The Haworth Press, Inc.) Vol. 6, No. 2, 2005, pp. 5-15; and: *Acute Reactions to Trauma and Psychotherapy: A Multidisciplinary and International Perspective* (ed: Etzel Cardeña, and Kristin Croyle) The Haworth Medical Press, an imprint of The Haworth Press, Inc., 2005, pp. 5-15. Single or multiple copies of this article are available for a fee from The Haworth Document Delivery Service [1-800-HAWORTH, 9:00 a.m. - 5:00 p.m. (EST). E-mail address: docdelivery@haworthpress.com].

Available online at http://www.haworthpress.com/web/JTD
© 2005 by The Haworth Press, Inc. All rights reserved.
doi:10.1300/J229v06n02_02

There is currently unprecedented attention on the means to identify people shortly after trauma who will develop chronic posttraumatic stress disorder (PTSD). This impetus has resulted, in part, from the desire to provide early interventions to people who are at risk of PTSD. This review will discuss recent attempts to identify acutely traumatized people who are at risk of PTSD, evaluate the predictive power of acute stress disorder (ASD), and suggest the likely areas for future developments in the pursuit of early prediction of PTSD.

## THE COURSE OF TRAUMA RESPONSES

Identifying people who are likely to develop PTSD has traditionally been a difficult task because most people experience marked stress reactions in the initial weeks after trauma exposure. Despite this initial stress, however, the majority of these people will adapt in the following months. For example, although in one study 70% of women and 50% of men were diagnosed with PTSD at an average of 19 days after an assault, the rate of PTSD at 4-month follow-up dropped to 21% for women and zero for men (Riggs, Rothbaum, & Foa, 1995). Similarly, whereas 94% of rape victims displayed PTSD symptoms two weeks post-trauma, this rate dropped to 47% eleven weeks later (Rothbaum, Foa, Riggs, Murdock, and Walsh, 1992). Similarly, half of a sample meeting criteria for PTSD following a motor vehicle accident (MVA) had remitted by six months and two-thirds had remitted by one year post-trauma (Blanchard et al., 1996). These results suggest that there is a need to identify particular reactions that distinguish between transient stress reactions and those initial reactions that will develop into chronic PTSD.

## ACUTE DISSOCIATION AND PTSD

A major theory guiding recent investigations of early predictors of chronic PTSD has involved the pivotal role of dissociation. This notion holds that dissociative reactions during or after trauma may lead to fragmented encoding and consolidation of trauma memories and their associated affect, and that this subsequently impedes emotional processing and resolution of the experience (Cardeña & Spiegel, 1993; Spiegel, Koopman, Cardeña, & Classen, 1996). This conceptualization of dissociation traces its historical roots to the work of Janet (1907), Prince (1905/1978), and Breuer and Freud (1895/1986).

A range of studies has reported that dissociative reactions at the time of the trauma are predictive of posttraumatic stress symptoms (Bremner & Brett, 1997; Holen, 1993; Koopman, Classen, & Spiegel, 1994; Marmar et al., 1994; McFarlane, 1986; Shalev, Orr, & Pitman, 1993; Shalev, Peri, Canetti, & Schreiber, 1996; Solomon & Mikulincer, 1992; Solomon, Mikulincer, & Benbenistry, 1989; Spiegel et al., 1996). For example, Holen (1993) found that peritraumatic dissociation in survivors of the North Sea oilrig disaster predicted subsequent adjustment. Similarly, Solomon et al. (1989) reported that numbing in the acute trauma phase accounted for 20% of the variance of subsequent PTSD. Ehlers, Mayou, and Bryant (1998) conducted a longitudinal study of patients who attended an emergency room after motor vehicle accidents, and reassessed them at three months and one year. This study found that chronic PTSD was associated with trauma severity, perceived threat, female gender, previous emotional problems, and dissociation during the trauma. Using a similar design, Shalev and colleagues assessed trauma survivors who presented at an emergency room, and re-assessed them one week, one month, and four months post-trauma (Shalev, Freedman, Peri, Brandes, Sahar, Orr, & Pitman, 1998). Although they did not report predictive power of acute symptoms, they found that individuals who subsequently developed PTSD and comorbid depression reported more peritraumatic dissociation than those who subsequently developed only PTSD, who in turn reported more dissociation than those with only depression or no disorder. In summary, there are initial indications that suggest a relationship between peritraumatic dissociation and PTSD.

There is evidence to suggest, however, that the reported relationship between acute dissociation and subsequent PTSD is more complex than has often been assumed. Whereas early dissociative responses have been linked to persistent PTSD in nonsexual assault victims, this relationship has not been observed in victims of rape (Dancu, Riggs, Hearst-Ikeda, Shoyer, & Foa, 1996). One investigation of ASD following motor vehicle accidents (MVAs) found that early dissociation was not indicative of poorer outcome at six months post-trauma; however, this study's inferences were limited by the assessment tools and the retrospective reporting of acute dissociation (Barton, Blanchard, & Hickling, 1996). Holen (1993) found that whereas peritraumatic reactions were predictive of the short-term outcome, they were less important in contributing to longer term adjustment. These findings suggest that the relationship between acute dissociation and longer-term psychopathology is not linear and is more complex than was initially suggested.

## ACUTE STRESS DISORDER

The acute stress disorder (ASD) diagnosis was introduced into the *DSM-IV* (American Psychiatric Association, 1994) to fill a diagnostic gap because the PTSD diagnosis did not address post-trauma symptoms experienced in the first month after trauma. Since the *DSM-III-R* (American Psychiatric Association, 1987), diagnosing PTSD within a month after the trauma was precluded because of concerns that this would pathologize transient stress reactions. An additional reason for the introduction of the ASD diagnosis was to identify acutely traumatized people who would develop chronic PTSD. An additional rationale for the ASD diagnosis was to recognize the pivotal role of dissociation in trauma response (Cardeña, Lews-Fernández, Beahr, Pakianathan, & Spiegel, 1996). The ASD diagnosis was influenced strongly by the proposition that dissociative reactions are a crucial mechanism in post-traumatic adjustment. To meet criteria for ASD one must have a fearful response to experiencing or witnessing a threatening event (Cluster A). The requisite symptoms to meet ASD include three dissociative symptoms (Cluster B), one reexperiencing symptom (Cluster C), marked avoidance (Cluster D), marked anxiety or increased arousal (Cluster E), and evidence of significant distress or impairment (Cluster F). The disturbance must last for a minimum of two days and a maximum of four weeks (Cluster G), after which time a diagnosis of PTSD should be considered. The primary difference between the criteria for ASD and PTSD is the former's emphasis on dissociative reactions to the trauma. The diagnosis of ASD requires that the individual has at least three of the following: (a) a subjective sense of numbing or detachment, (b) reduced awareness of one's surroundings, (c) derealization, (d) depersonalization, or (e) dissociative amnesia (for a review, see Bryant & Harvey, 2002).

Since the introduction of the diagnosis, there have been a number of longitudinal studies indexing the relationship between ASD and subsequent development of PTSD. In an initial study, Spiegel and colleagues prospectively studied 154 survivors of the 1991 Oakland/Berkeley firestorm (Spiegel et al., 1996). Using the Stanford Acute Stress Reaction Questionnaire (Cardeña, Classen, & Spiegel, 1991), survivors completed an inventory of dissociative and anxiety symptoms within three weeks of the fire and completed the Civilian Version of the Mississippi Scale for Posttraumatic Stress Disorder (Keane, Wolfe, & Taylor, 1987) and the Impact of Event Scale (Horowitz, Wilner, & Alvarez, 1979) seven months later. The authors calculated the sensitivity and specificity of each acute symptom in predicting a group of participants who at follow-up comprised the 18 people with the highest 5% on the psychopathology measures. Spiegel et al. (1996) observed that three dissociative symptoms combined with reexperiencing, avoidance, and arousal symptoms best predicted subsequent distress. This study was limited by not indexing subsequent PTSD diagnosis and the sample was not fully representative of the eligible population.

Since that initial study, 12 prospective studies have assessed the relationship between ASD in the initial month after trauma, and development of subsequent PTSD using prospective designs (Brewin et al., 1999; Bryant & Harvey, 1998; Creamer, O'Donnell, & Pattison, 2004; Difede et al., 2002; Harvey & Bryant, 1998a, 1999, 2000b; Holeva, Tarrier, & Wells, 2001; Kangas, Henry, & Bryant, 2005; Murray, Ehlers, & Mayou, 2002; Schnyder et al., 2001; Staab, Grieger, Fullerton, & Ursano, 1996). In terms of people who meet criteria for ASD, a number of studies have found that approximately three-quarters of trauma survivors who display ASD subsequently develop PTSD (Brewin et al., 1999; Bryant & Harvey, 1998; Difede et al., 2002; Harvey & Bryant, 1998a, 1999, 2000b; Holeva, Tarrier, & Wells, 2001; Kangas, Henry, & Bryant, 2005; Murray et al., 2002;). Relative to the expected remission of most people who display initial posttraumatic stress reactions, these studies indicate that the ASD diagnosis is performing reasonably well in predicting people who will develop PTSD.

The major weakness of the ASD diagnosis, however, is the general finding that many people develop PTSD without initially displaying ASD. In most studies, the minority of people who eventually developed PTSD initially met criteria for ASD. That is, whereas the majority of people who develop ASD are high risk for developing subsequent PTSD, there are many other people who will develop PTSD who do not initially meet ASD criteria. It appears that a major reason for people who are high risk for PTSD not meeting ASD criteria is the requirement that three dissociative symptoms be displayed. In one study, 60% of people who met all ASD criteria except for the dissociation cluster met PTSD criteria 6 months later (Harvey & Bryant, 1998a), and 75% of these people still had PTSD 2 years later (Harvey & Bryant, 1999b). It appears that emphasizing dissociation in formulae that attempt to predict subsequent PTSD leads to many people who will develop PTSD not being identified as high risk for PTSD development.

Overall, these initial studies provide partial support for the ASD diagnosis because they indicate that a significant proportion of people who initially meet criteria for ASD subsequently display persistent PTSD. It is important to note, however, that a significant proportion of people develop PTSD without initially satisfying ASD criteria. For example, Harvey and Bryant (1998) found that 60% of those who satisfied all ASD criteria except dissociation were diagnosed with PTSD six months post-trauma. The converging evidence suggests that the current emphasis on dissociative symptoms in the ASD definition needs to be questioned because a significant proportion of individuals who initially present with acute stress reactions that lack dissociative symptoms are also high risk for developing PTSD.

The finding that only a subset of people who develop PTSD initially display dissociative reactions can be explained by diathesis-stress models of dissociation. These models propose that whereas dissociative-prone individuals react to stress with dissociative symptoms, people who lack dissociative capacity will respond with non-dissociative symptoms (Butler, Duran, Jasiukaitis, Koopman, & Spiegel, 1996; Kihlstrom, Glisky, & Angiulo, 1994). This proposition is consistent with evidence that higher levels of hypnotizability have been reported in people with ASD compared to those who report a comparable acute stress reaction but lack dissociative symptoms (Bryant, Guthrie, & Moulds, 2001).

## ALTERNATIVES TO ACUTE STRESS DISORDER

If the ASD diagnosis is not optimal for predicting subsequent PTSD, what are the better alternatives? In terms of available data, there no particular symptoms that accurately predict the development of PTSD. It is important to note that the primary goal of symptoms is to differentiate between clinical presentations, and not to predict subsequent functioning. Accordingly, embodying risk factors within a diagnostic category may limit the potential for determining the optimal indicators of PTSD shortly after trauma. It seems likely that the most fruitful means of identifying early predictors of PTSD lies beyond symptoms or diagnostic categories.

Cognitive mechanisms, rather than symptoms, may be a useful means of enhancing prediction of PTSD. Recent cognitive models of PTSD have postulated that the appraisals that one makes of the traumatic event, the resulting symptoms, and one's capacity to cope is pivotal in the development and maintenance of PTSD (Ehlers & Clark, 2000). There is initial evidence that a catastrophic cognitive style in the initial period after trauma may contribute significantly to subsequent PTSD. People with ASD display more catastrophic beliefs about possible future harm (Smith & Bryant, 1999; Warda & Bryant, 1998).

Prospective analysis has found that negative appraisals three months after trauma predicts PTSD at one year (Ehlers et al., 1998). Similarly, catastrophic appraisals in the initial month are associated with chronic PTSD (Engelhard, van den Hout, Arntz, & McNally, 2002). It also appears that the attributions that people make about their trauma can influence subsequent PTSD. For example, there is evidence that people who attribute responsibility to another person in the acute phase are more likely to report PTSD twelve months later (Andrews, Brewin, Rose, & Kirk, 2000). It appears that the nature of the attributions is important, however, because a prospective study of crime victims found that the attributions of shame in the initial month predicted PTSD six months later (Delahanty et al., 1997). These data support the proposition that how people appraise their situation in the initial period is predictive of subsequent PTSD. The role of appraisals may also explain some of the mixed findings concerning the role of acute symptoms in predicting PTSD. For example, one person may experience emotional numbing and interpret this reaction as a sign that they are losing their sanity. Another person may simply attribute the experience of emotional numbing to the temporary shock of surviving a trauma. Whereas both individuals may have experienced the same symptom (i.e., emotional numbing), only the former person's reaction may contribute to a psychopathological reaction.

## FUTURE DIRECTIONS

There is a significant need for further prospective research to improve our understanding of the optimal predictors of PTSD. This research requires large representative populations. To date, most prospective studies have been restricted to samples of several hundred people. To adequately understand the relationship between acute reaction and the variety of responses that can occur following trauma, there is a need for studies involving thousands of participants. Further, these studies should investigate the range of potential predictors, including behavioral, cognitive, and biological reactions that may predict PTSD. Finally, it is important to identify early predictors of the array of posttraumatic disorders, including posttraumatic depression, substance abuse, and other conditions. It is apparent that acute dissociation is an important factor in the acute trauma response, but more rigorous research is required to delineate the exact role that dissociative responses may play in mediating subsequent psychiatric disorder. The potential clinical benefits of early intervention highlight the need for rigorous research that will identify factors with optimal sensitivity and specificity in predicting posttraumatic dysfunction.

## REFERENCES

American Psychiatric Association. (1987). *Diagnostic and statistical manual of mental disorders, 3rd ed., revised.* Washington, DC: Author.

American Psychiatric Association. (1994). *Diagnostic and statistical manual of mental disorders, 4th ed.* Washington, DC: Author.

Andrews, B., Brewin, C.R., Rose, S., & Kirk, M. (2000). Predicting PTSD in victims of violent crime: The role of shame, anger and blame. *Journal of Abnormal Psychology, 109,* 69-73.

Barton, K.A., Blanchard, E.B., & Hickling, E.J. (1996). Antecedents and consequences of acute stress disorder among motor vehicle accident victims. *Behaviour Research and Therapy, 34,* 805-813.

Blanchard, E.B., Hickling, E.J., Barton, K.A., Taylor, A.E., Loos, W.R., & Jones-Alexander, J. (1996). One-year prospective follow-up of motor vehicle accident victims. *Behaviour Research and Therapy, 34,* 775-786.

Bremner, J.D., & Brett, E. (1997). Trauma-related dissociative states and long-term psychopathology in posttraumatic stress disorder. *Journal of Traumatic Stress, 10,* 37-49.

Breuer, J., & Freud, S. (1895/1986). *Studies on hysteria.* New York: Basic Books (Original work published in 1895).

Brewin, C.R., Andrews, B., Rose, S., & Kirk, M. (1999). Acute stress disorder and posttraumatic stress disorder in victims of violent crime. *American Journal of Psychiatry, 156,* 360-365.

Bryant, R.A., & Harvey, A.G. (1998). Relationship of acute stress disorder and posttraumatic stress disorder following mild traumatic brain injury. *American Journal of Psychiatry, 155,* 625-629.

Bryant, R.A., Moulds, M., & Guthrie, R.M. (2000). Acute stress disorder scale: A self-report measure of acute stress disorder. *Psychological Assessment, 12,* 61-68.

Bryant, R.A., Guthrie, R.M., & Moulds, M.L. (2001). Hypnotizability in acute stress disorder. *American Journal of Psychiatry, 158,* 600-604.

Butler, L.D., Duran, R.E.F., Jasiukaitis, P., Koopman, C., & Spiegel, D. (1996). Hypnotizability and traumatic experience: A diathesis-stress model of dissociative symptomatology. *American Journal of Psychiatry, 153,* Suppl. 78, 42-63.

Cardeña, E., Lews-Fernández, R., Beahr, D., Pakianathan, I., & Spiegel, D. (1996). Dissociative disorders. In T.A. Widiger, A.J. Francis, H.J. Pincus, R. Ross, M.B. First, & W.W. Davis (Eds.), *Sourcebook for the DSM-IV, Vol. II* (pp. 973-1005). Washington, DC: American Psychiatric Press.

Cardeña, E., Koopman, C., Classen, C., Waelde, L.C., & Spiegel, D. (2000). Psychometric properties of the Stanford Acute Stress Reaction Questionnaire (SASRQ): A valid and reliable measure of acute stress. *Journal of Traumatic Stress, 13,* 719-734.

Cardeña, E., & Spiegel, D. (1993). Dissociative reactions to the San Francisco Bay Area earthquake of 1989. *American Journal of Psychiatry, 150,* 474-478.

Classen, C., Koopman, C., & Spiegel, D. (1993). Trauma and dissociation. *Bulletin of the Menninger Clinic, 57,* 178-194.

Creamer, M.C., O'Donnell, M.L., & Pattison, P. (2004). The relationship between acute stress disorder and posttraumatic stress disorder in severely injured trauma survivors. *Behaviour Research and Therapy, 42,* 315-328.

Dancu, C.V., Riggs, D.S., Hearst-Ikeda, D., Shoyer, B.G., & Foa, E.B. (1996). Dissociative experiences and posttraumatic stress disorder among female victims of criminal assault and rape. *Journal of Traumatic Stress, 9,* 253-267.

Delahanty, D.L., Herberman, H.B., Craig, K.J., Hayward, M.C., Fullerton, C.S., Ursano, R.J., & Baum, A. (1997). Acute and chronic distress and posttraumatic stress disorder as a function of responsibility for serious motor vehicle accidents. *Journal of Consulting and Clinical Psychology, 65,* 560-567.

Difede, J., Ptacek, J.T., Roberts, J.G., Barocas, D., Rives, W., Apfeldorf, W.J., & Yurt, R. (2002). Acute stress disorder after burn injury: A predictor of posttraumatic stress disorder. *Psychosomatic Medicine, 64,* 826-834.

Ehlers, A., & Clark, D. (2000). A cognitive model of posttraumatic stress disorder. *Behaviour Research and Therapy, 38,* 319-345.

Ehlers, A., Mayou, R.A., & Bryant, B. (1998). Psychological predictors of chronic PTSD after motor vehicle accidents. *Journal of Abnormal Psychology, 107,* 508-519.

Engelhard, I.M., van den Hout, M.A., Arntz, A., & McNally, R.J. (2002). A longitudinal study of "intrusion-based reasoning" and posttraumatic stress disorder after exposure to a train disaster. *Behaviour Research and Therapy, 40,* 1415-1424.

Harvey, A.G., & Bryant, R.A. (1998). Relationship of acute stress disorder and posttraumatic stress disorder following motor vehicle accidents. *Journal of Consulting and Clinical Psychology, 66,* 507-512.

Harvey, A.G., & Bryant, R.A. (1999). Relationship of acute stress disorder and posttraumatic stress disorder: A two-year prospective study. *Journal of Consulting and Clinical Psychology, 67,* 985-988.

Harvey, A.G., & Bryant, R.A. (2000). A two-year prospective evaluation of the relationship between acute stress disorder and posttraumatic stress disorder following mild traumatic brain injury. *American Journal of Psychiatry, 157,* 626-628.

Harvey, A.G., & Bryant, R.A. (2002). Acute stress disorder: A synthesis and critique. *Psychological Bulletin, 128,* 886-902.

Holen, A. (1993). The North Sea oil rig disaster. In J.P. Wilson & B. Raphael (Eds.), *International handbook of traumatic stress syndromes* (pp. 471-478). New York: Plenum.

Holeva, V., Tarrier, N., & Wells, A. (2001). Prevalence and predictors of acute stress disorder and PTSD following road traffic accidents: Thought control strategies and social support. *Behavior Therapy, 32,* 65-83.

Horowitz, M.J., Wilner, N., & Alvarez, W. (1979). The impact of event scale: A measure of subjective stress. *Psychosomatic Medicine, 41,* 209-218.

Janet, P. (1907). *The major symptoms of hysteria.* New York: McMillan.

Kangas, M., Henry, J.L., & Bryant, R.A. (2005). The relationship between acute stress disorder and posttraumatic stress disorder following cancer. *Journal of Consulting and Clinical Psychology, 73,* 360-364.

Keane, T.M., Wolfe, J., & Taylor, K.L. (1987). Post-traumatic stress disorder: Evidence for diagnostic validity and methods of psychological assessment. *Journal of Clinical Psychology, 43,* 32-43.

Kihlstrom, J. F., Glisky, M. L., & Angiulo, M. J. (1994). Dissociative tendencies and dissociative disorders. *Journal of Abnormal Psychology, 103,* 117-124.

Koopman, C., Classen, C., & Spiegel, D. (1994). Predictors of posttraumatic stress symptoms among survivors of the Oakland/Berkeley, California, firestorm. *American Journal of Psychiatry, 151,* 888-894.

Marmar, C.R., Weiss, D.S., Schlenger, W.E., Fairbank, J.A., Jordan, K., Kulka, R.A., & Hough, R.L. (1994). Peritraumatic dissociation and posttraumatic stress in male Vietnam theater veterans. *American Journal of Psychiatry, 151,* 902-907.

McFarlane, A.C. (1986). Posttraumatic morbidity of a disaster. *Journal of Nervous and Mental Disease, 174,* 4-14.

Murray, J., Ehlers, A., & Mayou, R.A. (2002). Dissociation and post-traumatic stress disorder: Two prospective studies of road traffic accident survivors. *British Journal of Psychiatry, 180,* 363-368.

Prince, M. (1905/1978). *The dissociation of a personality.* New York: Oxford University Press (Original work published in 1905).

Riggs, D.S., Rothbaum, B.O., & Foa, E.B. (1995). A prospective examination of symptoms of posttraumatic stress disorder in victims of nonsexual assault. *Journal of Interpersonal Violence, 10,* 201-213.

Rothbaum, B., Foa, E., Riggs, D., Murdock, T., & Walsh, W. (1992). A prospective examination of post-traumatic stress disorder in rape victims. *Journal of Traumatic Stress, 5,* 455-475.

Schnyder, U., Moergeli, H., Klaghofer, R., & Buddeberg, C. (2001). Incidence and prediction of posttraumatic stress disorder symptoms in severely injured accident victims. *American Journal of Psychiatry, 158,* 594-599.

Shalev, A.Y., Freedman, S., Peri, T., Brandes, D., & Sahar, T. (1997). Predicting PTSD in trauma survivors: Prospective evaluation of self-report and clinician administered instruments. *British Journal of Psychiatry, 170,* 558-564.

Shalev, A.Y., Orr, S.P., & Pitman, R.K. (1993). Psychophysiologic assessment of traumatic imagery in Israeli civilian patients with posttraumatic stress disorder. *American Journal of Psychiatry, 150,* 620-624.

Shalev, A.Y., Peri, T., Canetti, L., & Schreiber, S. (1996). Predictors of PTSD in injured trauma survivors: A prospective study. *American Journal of Psychiatry, 153,* 219-225.

Solomon, Z., & Mikulincer, M. (1992). Aftermaths of combat stress reactions: A three-year study. *British Journal of Clinical Psychology, 31,* 21-32.

Solomon, Z., Mikulincer, M., & Benbenishty, R. (1989). Combat stress reactions: Clinical manifestations and correlates. *Military Psychology, 1,* 35-47.

Spiegel, D., Koopman, C., Cardeña, E., & Classen, C. (1996). Dissociative symptoms in the diagnosis of acute stress disorder. In L.K. Michelson & W.J. Ray (Eds.), *Handbook of dissociation: Theoretical, empirical, and clinical perspectives* (pp. 367-380). New York: Plenum Press.

Staab, J.P., Grieger, T.A., Fullerton, C.S., & Ursano, R.J. (1996). Acute stress disorder, subsequent posttraumatic stress disorder and depression after a series of typhoons. *Anxiety, 2,* 219-225.

# Aspects of Exposure in Childhood Trauma:
# The Stressor Criterion

Betty Pfefferbaum, MD, JD

**SUMMARY.** Attention to posttraumatic stress disorder (PTSD) in children has lagged behind the understanding of this disorder in adults. This article provides a brief review related to the stressor criterion of PTSD in children. The stressor criterion for PTSD includes three elements–an event, exposure, and a subjective reaction–each of which is described in the diagnostic criteria for the disorder. A host of stressors, both natural and human-caused, have the potential to evoke symptoms. Exposure can be direct–through, for example, physical presence, direct victimization, and witnessing, or indirect–through, for example, an interpersonal relationship with a direct victim. Exposure to media coverage of an event as a stressor for PTSD has also been examined. The requirement of a sub-

---

Betty Pfefferbaum is the Paul and Ruth Jonas Chair, Professor and Chairman, Department of Psychiatry and Behavioral Sciences, College of Medicine, University of Oklahoma Health Sciences Center, Oklahoma City, OK.

Address correspondence to: Betty Pfefferbaum, MD, JD, Department of Psychiatry and Behavioral Sciences, College of Medicine, University of Oklahoma Health Sciences Center, 920 Stanton L. Young Boulevard., WP-3470, Oklahoma City, OK 73104 (E-mail: betty-pfefferbaum@ouhsc.edu).

This review was supported under Award Number MIPT106-113-2000-020 from the Oklahoma City National Memorial Institute for the Prevention of Terrorism and the Office for Domestic Preparedness, U.S. Department of Homeland Security. Points of view in this document are those of the author and do not necessarily represent the official position of the Oklahoma City National Memorial Institute for the Prevention of Terrorism or the U.S. Department of Homeland Security.

[Haworth co-indexing entry note]: "Aspects of Exposure in Childhood Trauma: The Stressor Criterion." Pfefferbaum, Betty. Co-published simultaneously in *Journal of Trauma & Dissociation* (The Haworth Medical Press, an imprint of The Haworth Press, Inc.) Vol. 6, No. 2, 2005, pp. 17-26; and: *Acute Reactions to Trauma and Psychotherapy: A Multidisciplinary and International Perspective* (ed: Etzel Cardeña, and Kristin Croyle) The Haworth Medical Press, an imprint of The Haworth Press, Inc., 2005, pp. 17-26. Single or multiple copies of this article are available for a fee from The Haworth Document Delivery Service [1-800-HAWORTH, 9:00 a.m. - 5:00 p.m. (EST). E-mail address: docdelivery@haworthpress.com].

jective reaction to the event is supported by research. A number of factors limit the ability to investigate issues associated with the stressor criterion including difficulty obtaining reliable and valid measures. Future studies should focus on specific aspects of exposure and outcomes, indirect forms of exposure, the clinical significance of findings, and the various factors that influence a child's reaction to trauma. *[Article copies available for a fee from The Haworth Document Delivery Service: 1-800-HAWORTH. E-mail address: <docdelivery@haworthpress.com> Website: <http://www.HaworthPress.com> © 2005 by The Haworth Press, Inc. All rights reserved.]*

**KEYWORDS.** Stressor, posttraumatic stress disorder, PTSD

Conditions consistent with posttraumatic stress disorder (PTSD) have been described for thousands of years. The disorder first appeared by the name post-traumatic stress disorder in the third edition of the *Diagnostic and Statistical Manual* (*DSM-III*; American Psychiatric Association (APA), 1980). Like with many disorders, attention to PTSD in children lagged behind that in adults with age-specific features first appearing in revised third edition of the *Diagnostic and Statistical Manual* (*DSM-III-R*; American Psychiatric Association, 1987).

Exposure and response to the stressor constitute the first criterion for PTSD-Criterion A, the stressor criterion. The stressor criterion has been called the "gatekeeper" of PTSD (Davidson & Foa, 1991); without exposure to a stressor, the diagnosis is not even considered. The stressor criterion has been closely scrutinized, as have all of the PTSD criteria. The first question of interest is what qualifies as a stressor and what constitutes exposure. Both *DSM-III* (APA, 1980) and *DSM-III-R* (APA, 1987) required the event to be "outside the range of usual human experience" (APA, 1980, p. 236; APA, 1987, p. 250). The fourth edition of the *Diagnostic and Statistical Manual* (*DSM-IV*; APA, 1994) qualified more common events as stressors, but required them to be "extreme" (p. 424). While *DSM-III* was silent on what constituted exposure, *DSM-III-R* began to explicate what might qualify including "serious threat or harm" to relatives or friends, "seeing another person who has recently been, or is being, seriously injured or killed," or "learning about a serious threat or harm to a close friend or relative" (APA, 1987, pp. 247-48). *DSM-IV* further qualified exposure by adding the subjective component of "intense fear, helplessness, or horror" (APA, 1994, p. 428).

*DSM-IV* set out two elements of exposure. The first element of Criterion A is exposure that can take the form of experiencing, witnessing, or confronting an event or events involving "actual or threatened death or serious injury, or a threat to the physical integrity of self or others" (p. 427). The second element of Criterion A requires that the individual respond with "intense fear, helplessness, or horror" (p. 428). These modifications in diagnostic criteria invite discussion and research to clarify the importance of each aspect of this criterion-the event, exposure, and peritraumatic reaction. This article provides a brief review of the literature related to the stressor criterion in children.

## THE TRAUMATIC EVENT

A host of stressors, both natural and human-caused, have the potential to evoke symptoms. Naturally occurring stressors include, for example, tornadoes, earthquakes, and medical illnesses. Human-caused events include accidents, domestic and community violence, murder, terrorism, and war. Some of these are singular events; others involve chronic or repeated exposure. Trauma exposure appears to be common in children. More than two-fifths of adolescents in a community sample had at least one experience that could meet the stressor criterion of *DSM-III-R* trauma by the age of 18 years (Giaconia et al., 1995).

Different types of stressors may be associated with different reactions (March, 1993; McCloskey & Walker, 2000), though this issue is difficult to study because many factors influence a child's response including magnitude and severity of the stressor (March, 1993), aspects of exposure, characteristics of the child and family, and aspects of the recovery environment (Pfefferbaum, 2002). Human-caused events are thought to be more traumatizing than natural ones (APA, 1980, 1987, 1994). Death of a loved one is particularly traumatizing for children. McCloskey and Walker (2000) found the death or illness of someone close to a child to be more likely than family violence, violent crime, or accidents to precipitate PTSD in children. Stoppelbein and Greening (2000) found that children who had lost a parent to an illness or accident endorsed more PTSD symptoms than either children exposed to a fatal tornado or non-traumatized children. Of the bereaved children, female sex, younger age, and PTSD symptoms in the surviving parent were associated with risk.

## EXPOSURE

The *DSM-IV* (APA, 1994) describes both direct and indirect exposure in the diagnosis of PTSD. Exposure takes many forms including physical presence, direct victimization, and witnessing or confronting an event experienced by a family member or close associate (APA, 1994). Intensity and duration of exposure are likely to influence outcome, and repeated or chronic exposure may be more traumatizing than a single event or exposure that is time-limited (March, 1993).

### Direct Exposure

A number of studies have demonstrated the role of physical proximity in the trauma response and a dose-response relationship between exposure and symptomatology (Breton, Valla, & Lambert, 1993; March, Amaya-Jackson, Terry, & Costanzo, 1997; Pynoos et al., 1987). This dose effect may not be prominent when other factors, such as extensive interpersonal exposure (through relationship to direct victims) and media coverage, characterize the disaster (Tyano et al., 1996). Physical injury resulting from a traumatic event may relate to symptom development. Daviss, Mooney and colleagues (2000) found that 12.5% of children hospitalized for accidental injuries developed PTSD and another 16.7% developed subsyndromal PTSD.

### Interpersonal Exposure

Interpersonal exposure is a form of indirect exposure that occurs through relationship to direct victims (APA, 1994; McCloskey & Walker, 2000; Pfefferbaum, Nixon, Krug et al., 1999; Pfefferbaum, Nixon, Tucker et al., 1999). The closeness of the relationship between the child and victim may influence the child's response (Pfefferbaum, Nixon, Krug et al., 1999; Pfefferbaum, Nixon, Tucker et al., 1999), with closer relationships resulting in heightened trauma responses.

### Indirect and Distant Trauma

Although the use of the term "confronted" in the *DSM-IV* (APA, 1994, p. 427) criteria for PTSD is less than clear on intent, the accompanying text appears to define it and limit it to a form of exposure to events experienced by "a family member or other close associate" (p. 424). Terr and colleagues (1999) have proposed a broader "spectrum PTSD" classification for indirect trauma. They examined children's responses to the 1986 Challenger space shuttle explosion resulting from three forms of perceptual exposure–observing the launch directly from the viewing stands, watching it live on television, and hearing about it later, and from three levels of interpersonal involvement–personal relationship with the teacher on the flight, residence in the same geographic region but not students of the teacher, and residence on the West Coast with no relationship to the teacher. The spectrum classification includes distant trauma (reaction to a real event observed at the time but from a distant safe site), close call (near miss), indirect trauma (reaction to an event not directly observable), vicarious trauma (reaction to a highly threatening event that was not directly observable but was nationally threatening), mass threat (reaction to a pending or possible national or worldwide event), mass hysteria (reaction to a nonspecific threat with acquisition of symptoms through social means), and copycatting (imitation of symptoms transmitted through social means).

Although the *DSM-IV* (APA, 1994) appears to preclude the application of the PTSD diagnosis to those whose only exposure is through the media, studies have found an association between exposure to media coverage and PTSD reactions (Pfefferbaum, Nixon, Krug et al., 1999; Pfefferbaum, Nixon, Tucker et al., 1999; Schuster et al., 2001). This was examined in relation to the coverage of the Oklahoma City bombing (Pfefferbaum, Nixon, Krug et al., 1999; Pfefferbaum, Nixon, Tucker et al., 1999) and the September 11 terrorist attacks (Schuster et al., 2001). In some instances, like these incidents, it may be impossible to distinguish symptoms related to the event itself and those related to media coverage. In fact, media coverage may constitute the primary source of exposure for many persons. Other types of events raise similar concern. For example, evacuation notices (Breton et al., 1993; Handford et al., 1986) and disaster warnings (Kiser et al., 1993) have been implicated as potential trauma-inducing experiences. But, while media coverage conveys the message, it may not be the coverage per se, but anticipation or knowledge of the event that constitutes the stressor.

Extent of exposure to coverage of an incident may be associated with symptom development (Pfefferbaum, Nixon, Krug et al., 1999; Pfefferbaum et al., 2001). Nader and colleagues (1993) found that television viewing contributed to PTSD symptomatology even after controlling for the effects of other forms of exposure in Kuwaiti children following the Gulf War. Exposure to television coverage of the Oklahoma City bombing had a small but significant effect in relationship to PTSD reactions in indirectly exposed children in Oklahoma City (Pfefferbaum, Nixon,

Tucker et al., 1999; Pfefferbaum et al., 2001). According to parent reports, children watched television coverage of the September 11 terrorist attacks for a mean of 3.0 hours on the day of the attacks. Approximately one-third of parents tried to prevent or limit their children's viewing. Parents of children who were perceived as stressed were more likely than other parents to restrict their children's exposure. For children whose viewing was not restricted, hours of viewing were related to the number of stress symptoms (Schuster et al., 2001).

## Multiple Forms of Exposure

Traumatized children commonly experience multiple forms of exposure such as physical proximity and relationship to direct victims. This may increase risk for symptom development. March and colleagues (1997) found greatest risk for PTSD symptomatology associated with combined physical and interpersonal exposure.

Studies have examined the relative impact or interactions among various forms of exposure (March et al., 1997; McCloskey & Walker, 2000; Nader et al., 1993; Saigh, 1991), but the results of these studies vary. Saigh (1991) found no statistically significant differences in the PTSD reactions of Lebanese children stemming from four types of exposure to war-related trauma-direct experience, observation, verbal mediation, and combinations of these. In a study of Kuwaiti children during the Gulf War, PTSD symptomatology correlated positively with direct exposure through witnessing, and with indirect exposure through television coverage of war trauma, but not with indirect exposure through interpersonal relationships (Nader et al., 1993). Sack and colleagues (1996) studied the effects of multiple trauma in adolescents exposed to war, resettlement, and stressful life events. A diagnosis of PTSD was strongly associated with war trauma; resettlement stress was more intense in those with PTSD; depression was more related to recent stresses.

## Secondary Adversities and Traumatic Reminders

Traumatic events do not occur in isolation, and secondary adversities and traumatic reminders may trigger or intensify symptoms. Secondary adversities include displacement and relocation, property and economic loss, family and social problems, and disrupted interpersonal support networks (Laor et al., 1996; Najarian, Goenjian, Pelcovitz, Mandel, & Najarian, 1996; Sack, Clarke, & Seeley, 1996; Shaw et al., 1995). Studies have examined symptomatology in evacuated, displaced, or resettled children (Breton et al., 1993; Laor et al., 1996; Najarian et al., 1996; Sack et al., 1996), but have not isolated the specific aspect of these experiences that is related to PTSD symptoms. Traumatic reminders–stimulus cues that activate symptoms–may also interfere with recovery (Pynoos, 1996; Shaw et al., 1995), and formerly neutral or positive cues may become distressing through association with the traumatic experience (Pynoos, 1996).

## SUBJECTIVE REACTION

Current *DSM-IV* diagnostic criteria include a subjective response to exposure (APA, 1994), which was absent from the *DSM-III* (APA, 1980) and *DSM-III-R* (APA, 1987). This subjective response to the stressor is characterized as "intense fear, helplessness, or horror," (APA, 1994, p. 428). Research supports its inclusion in the criteria (Lonigan, Shannon, Taylor, Finch, & Sallee, 1994; Pfefferbaum, Nixon, Tucker et al., 1999). Green and colleagues (1991) found life threat the most powerful predictor of PTSD in child victims of the Buffalo Dam disaster. Emotions, such as sadness, worry, fear, and loneliness during a traumatic event, may also predict later symptomatology (Lonigan et al., 1994).

The *DSM-IV* (APA, 1994) criteria for acute stress disorder emphasize the importance of peritraumatic dissociation, which, except in trauma associated with sexual abuse, has received relatively little attention in children (Carrion & Steiner, 2000; Daviss, Racusin et al., 2000; Perry, Pollard, Blakley, Baker, & Vigilante, 1995). Many parents reported that their children, hospitalized for injuries, experienced dissociative symptoms, with almost 20% meeting the full dissociative criterion for acute distress disorder (Daviss, Racusin et al., 2000). Carrion and Steiner (2000) found a modest relationship between trauma and dissociation in a sample of delinquent adolescents and support for an association of history of physical abuse and neglect with dissociation.

## IMPLICATIONS AND FUTURE DIRECTIONS

There are methodological difficulties in obtaining reliable and valid measures of exposure and initial subjective reactions that must be addressed. Aspects of exposure are typically measured by retrospective self-report, yet a number of factors, which have not been well examined, potentially influence recall of trauma (Pynoos, 1996). Future studies should be designed to address specific aspects of exposure and outcomes. For example, while many studies examine the role of exposure in symptom response, a number of specific aspects of exposure have not been well explored. Of great interest, particularly with the advent of major terrorist events in this country, are indirect forms of exposure and the PTSD spectrum. The impact of exposure has been measured primarily in relation to PTSD symptoms or reactions, potentially obscuring important differences between normal reactions and those that have clinical significance. Therefore, a second issue that warrants further exploration is the distinction between PTSD diagnosis and symptoms, important especially with regard to functioning and prognosis. The child's subjective response is central to our understanding of the post-trauma process and course of recovery, the relationship between the biology and psychology of the disease, the relative importance of specific symptoms, and treatment planning. Finally, the child's emotional response to a traumatic event or experience does not depend on exposure alone. A host of individual, family, and social factors influence the relationship and must be considered in the context of exposure in both clinical practice and research.

# REFERENCES

American Psychiatric Association (1980). *Diagnostic and statistical manual of mental disorders, 3rd ed.* Washington, DC: Author.

American Psychiatric Association (1987). *Diagnostic and statistical manual of mental disorders, 3rd ed., revised.* Washington, DC: Author.

American Psychiatric Association (1994). *Diagnostic and statistical manual of mental disorders, 4th ed.* Washington, DC: Author.

Breton, J.J., Valla, J.P., & Lambert, J. (1993). Industrial disaster and mental health of children and their parents. *Journal of the American Academy of Child and Adolescent Psychiatry, 32,* 438-445.

Carrion, V.G., & Steiner, H. (2000). Trauma and dissociation in delinquent adolescents. *Journal of the American Academy of Child and Adolescent Psychiatry, 39,* 353-359.

Davidson, J.R.T., & Foa, E.B. (1991). Diagnostic issues in posttraumatic stress disorder: Considerations for the *DSM-IV. Journal of Abnormal Psychology, 100,* 346-355.

Daviss, W.B., Mooney, D., Racusin, R., Ford, J.D., Fleischer, A., & McHugo, G.J. (2000). Predicting posttraumatic stress after hospitalization for pediatric injury. *Journal of the American Academy of Child and Adolescent Psychiatry, 39,* 576-583.

Daviss, W.B., Racusin, R., Fleischer, A., Mooney, D., Ford, J.D., & McHugo, G.J. (2000). Acute stress disorder symptomatology during hospitalization for pediatric injury. *Journal of the American Academy of Child and Adolescent Psychiatry, 39,* 569-575.

Giaconia, R.M., Reinherz, H.Z., Silverman, A.B., Pakiz, B., Frost, A.K., & Cohen, E. (1995). Traumas and posttraumatic stress disorder in a community population of older adolescents. *Journal of the American Academy of Child and Adolescent Psychiatry, 34,* 1369-1380.

Green, B.L., Korol, M., Grace, M.C., Vary, M.G., Leonard, A.C., Gleser, G.C., & Smitson-Cohen, S. (1991). Children and disaster: Age, gender, and parental effects on PTSD symptoms. *Journal of the American Academy of Child and Adolescent Psychiatry, 30,* 945-951.

Handford, H.A., Mayes, S.D., Mattison, R.E., Humphrey, F.J., II, Bagnato, S., Bixler, E.O., & Kales, J.D. (1986). Child and parent reaction to the Three Mile Island nuclear accident. *Journal of the American Academy of Child Psychiatry, 25,* 346-356.

Kiser, L., Heston, J., Hickerson, S., Millsap, P., Nunn, W., & Pruitt, D. (1993). Anticipatory stress in children and adolescents. *American Journal of Psychiatry, 150,* 87-92.

Laor, N., Wolmer, L., Mayes, L.C., Golomb, A., Silverberg, D.S., Weizman, R., & Cohen, D.J. (1996). Israeli preschoolers under Scud missile attacks: A developmental perspective on risk-modifying factors. *Archives of General Psychiatry, 53,* 416-423.

Lonigan, C.J., Shannon, M.P., Taylor, C.M., Finch, A.J., Jr., & Sallee, F.R. (1994). Children exposed to disaster: II. Risk factors for the development of post-traumatic symptomatology. *Journal of the American Academy of Child and Adolescent Psychiatry, 33,* 94-105.

March, J.S. (1993). What constitutes a stressor? The "Criterion A" issue. In J.R.T. Davidson, & E.B. Foa (eds.), *Posttraumatic Stress Disorder: DSM-IV and beyond* (pp. 37-54). Washington, DC: American Psychiatric Press.

March, J.S., Amaya-Jackson, L., Terry, R., & Costanzo, P. (1997). Posttraumatic symptomatology in children and adolescents after an industrial fire. *Journal of the American Academy of Child and Adolescent Psychiatry, 36,* 1080-1088.

McCloskey, L.A., & Walker, M. (2000). Posttraumatic stress in children exposed to family violence and single-event trauma. *Journal of the American Academy of Child and Adolescent Psychiatry, 39,* 108-115.

Nader, K.O., Pynoos, R.S., Fairbanks, L.A., Al-Ajeel, M., & Al-Asfour, A. (1993). A preliminary study of PTSD and grief among the children of Kuwait following the Gulf crisis. *British Journal of Clinical Psychology, 32,* 407-416.

Najarian, L.M., Goenjian, A.K., Pelcovitz, D., Mandel, F., & Najarian, B. (1996). Relocation after a disaster: Posttraumatic stress disorder in Armenia after the earthquake. *Journal of the American Academy of Child and Adolescent Psychiatry, 35,* 374-383.

Perry, B.D., Pollard, R.A., Blakley, T.L., Baker, W.L., & Vigilante, D. (1995). Childhood trauma, the neurobiology of adaptation, and "use-dependent" development of the brain: How "states" become "traits." *Infant Mental Health Journal, 16,* 271-291.

Pfefferbaum, B. (2002). Posttraumatic stress disorder. In M. Lewis, (ed.), *Child and adolescent psychiatry*, (3rd ed.) (pp. 912-925). Philadelphia: Lippincott, Williams & Wilkins.

Pfefferbaum, B., Nixon, S.J., Krug, R.S., Tivis, R.D., Moore, V.L., Brown, J.M., Pynoos, R.S., Foy, D., & Gurwitch, R.H. (1999). Clinical needs assessment of middle and high school students following the 1995 Oklahoma City bombing. *American Journal of Psychiatry, 156,* 1069-1074.

Pfefferbaum, B., Nixon, S.J., Tivis, R.D., Doughty, D.E., Pynoos, R.S., Gurwitch, R.H., & Foy, D.W. (2001). Television exposure in children after a terrorist incident. *Psychiatry, 64,* 202-211.

Pfefferbaum, B., Nixon, S.J., Tucker, P.M., Tivis, R.D., Moore, V.L., Gurwitch, R.H., Pynoos, R.S., & Geis, H.K. (1999). Posttraumatic stress responses in bereaved children after the Oklahoma City bombing. *Journal of the American Academy of Child and Adolescent Psychiatry, 38,* 1372-1379.

Pynoos, R.S. (1996). Exposure to catastrophic violence and disaster in childhood. In C.R. Pfeffer, (Ed.), *Severe stress and mental disturbance in children* (pp. 181-208). Washington, DC: American Psychiatric Press, Inc.

Pynoos, R.S., Frederick, C., Nader, K., Arroyo, W., Steinberg, A., Eth, S., Nunez, F., & Fairbanks, L. (1987). Life threat and posttraumatic stress in school-age children. *Archives of General Psychiatry, 44,* 1057-1063.

Sack, W.H., Clarke, G.N., & Seeley, J. (1996). Multiple forms of stress in Cambodian adolescent refugees. *Child Development, 67,* 107-116.

Saigh, P.A. (1991). The development of posttraumatic stress disorder following four different types of traumatization. *Behaviour Research Therapy, 29,* 213-216.

Schuster, M.A., Stein, B.D., Jaycox, L.H., Collins, R.L., Marshall, G.N., Elliott, M.N., Zhou, A.J., Kanouse, D.E., Morrison, J.L., & Berry, S.H. (2001). A national survey of stress reactions after the September 11, 2001, terrorist attacks. *New England Journal of Medicine, 345,* 1507-1512.

Shaw, J.A., Applegate, B., Tanner, S., Perez, D., Rothe, E., Campo-Bowen, A.E., & Lahey, B.L. (1995). Psychological effects of Hurricane Andrew on an elementary school population. *Journal of the American Academy of Child and Adolescent Psychiatry, 34,* 1185-1192.

Stoppelbein, L., & Greening, L. (2000). Posttraumatic stress symptoms in parentally bereaved children and adolescents. *Journal of the American Academy of Child and Adolescent Psychiatry, 39,* 1112-1119.

Terr, L.C., Bloch, D.A., Michel, B.A., Shi, H., Reinhardt, J.A., & Metayer, S. (1999). Children's symptoms in the wake of Challenger: A field study of distant-traumatic effects and an outline of related conditions. *American Journal of Psychiatry, 156,* 1536-1544.

Tyano, S., Iancu, I., Solomon, Z., Sever, J., Goldstein, I., Touviana, Y., & Bleich, A. (1996). Seven-year follow-up of child survivors of a bus-train collision. *Journal of the American Academy of Child and Adolescent Psychiatry, 35,* 365-373.

# The Oklahoma City Bombing Study and Methodological Issues in Longitudinal Disaster Mental Health Research

Carol S. North, MD, MPE

**SUMMARY.** Several methodological issues may affect the findings of studies of the mental health effects of disasters over time. These issues include analysis of the course of individual disorders over time that may be lost when they are presented embedded in general summary statistics, consideration of assessment of psychiatric disorders versus symptoms, adherence to established criteria in assigning psychiatric diagnoses, and orientation of mental health issues to the type of disaster exposure of the sample. This report will explore these methodological issues in a review of disaster literature and in data obtained from study of survivors of the Oklahoma City bombing. Clinical implications of the data obtained from the Oklahoma City bombing study of survivors of the direct bomb blast are presented in the context of these methodological concerns. *[Article copies available for a fee from The Haworth Document Delivery Service: 1-800-HAWORTH. E-mail address: <docdelivery@haworthpress.com> Website: <http://www.HaworthPress.com> © 2005 by The Haworth Press, Inc. All rights reserved.]*

---

Carol S. North is affiliated with the Department of Psychiatry, Washington University School of Medicine, St. Louis, MO.

Address correspondence to: Carol S. North, MD, MPE, Department of Psychiatry, Washington University School of Medicine, 660 South Euclid Avenue, Campus Box 8134, St. Louis, MO 63110 (E-mail: NorthC@psychiatry.wustl.edu).

[Haworth co-indexing entry note]: "The Oklahoma City Bombing Study and Methodological Issues in Longitudinal Disaster Mental Health Research." North, Carol S. Co-published simultaneously in *Journal of Trauma & Dissociation* (The Haworth Medical Press, an imprint of The Haworth Press, Inc.) Vol. 6, No. 2, 2005, pp. 27-35; and: *Acute Reactions to Trauma and Psychotherapy: A Multidisciplinary and International Perspective* (ed: Etzel Cardeña, and Kristin Croyle) The Haworth Medical Press, an imprint of The Haworth Press, Inc., 2005, pp. 27-35. Single or multiple copies of this article are available for a fee from The Haworth Document Delivery Service [1-800-HAWORTH, 9:00 a.m. - 5:00 p.m. (EST). E-mail address: docdelivery@ haworthpress.com].

doi:10.1300/J229v06n02_04

**KEYWORDS.** Oklahoma City bombing, posttraumatic stress disorder, methodology

Clinicians working with survivors in early post-disaster settings have a need to project longer-term outcomes. Existing longitudinal group summary data from studies of disasters and terrorism demonstrate that posttraumatic stress disorder (PTSD) tends to diminish over time (Grace, Green, Lindy, & Leonard, 1993; Groenjian et al., 2000; Ursano, Fullerton, Kao, & Bhartiya, 1995; Weisaeth, 1985). Data presentation in longitudinal group summary format tracks group trends over time but could potentially mask within-individual changes embedded in the data. No specific information is provided on emergence of new cases or disappearance of symptomatology from initial assessment to follow-up.

Studies that have considered the temporal course of PTSD within individual survivors of disasters (Epstein, Fullerton, & Ursano, 1998; Grace et al., 1993; Groenjian et al., 2000; Johnson, North, & Smith, 2002; McFarlane, 1988; North, Smith, & Spitznagel, 1997; Steinglass & Gerrity, 1990; Wang et al., 2000; Weisaeth, 1985) and intentional human acts of mass violence (Abenhaim, 1992; Amir, Weil, Kaplan, Tocker, & Witztum, 1998; Curran et al., 1990; North et al., 1999; North, McCutcheon, Spitznagel, & Smith, 2002; Shalev, 1992) have provided evidence that the course of PTSD over time is not all unidirectional, with some cases recovering between baseline and follow-up, and others first being detected only later. Therefore, temporal comparisons within individuals demonstrate bidirectional dimensionality not possible in presentation of overall summary data on rates of disorders or group means at two time points.

Previous studies have provided little detail on the specific aspects of PTSD driving changes in outcomes over time. Several studies have provided indirect evidence of both late emergence of newly identified cases and disappearance of active psychopathology at follow-up, inferred through observation that combined rates of PTSD from both assessments are higher than the rates at either assessment alone. More information is needed about what these intra-individual changes represent, whether the cases identified only late indicate actual delayed-onset PTSD and whether the baseline cases not identified at follow-up represent truly recovered cases. Additional detail is desired on which aspects of the diagnostic criteria are critical in determining changes in diagnosis over time.

Other methodological issues reviewed in this report that may affect reported rates of PTSD and its apparent recovery as well as treatment needs include consideration of assessment of psychiatric disorders or symptoms, adherence to established criteria in assigning psychiatric diagnoses, and orientation of mental health outcomes to the type of disaster exposure of the sample.

To address these issues, this report examines baseline and follow-up data from a longitudinal study of the Oklahoma City bombing. In the Oklahoma City bombing study (North et al., 1999), 182 directly exposed survivors of the direct bomb blast, randomly selected from the Oklahoma Health Department's list of survivors with 71% participation, were interviewed using a structured diagnostic interview an average of six months after the disaster. A follow-up study was completed nearly a year later (75% re-interview at 17 months post-bombing) using the same assessment tools. This consistency of methods from baseline to follow-up allows comparison of findings and attribution of differences to temporal influences rather than inconsistencies in the assessment process.

## FINDINGS FROM THE OKLAHOMA CITY BOMBING STUDY

The baseline study of the Oklahoma City bombing found that 34% of participants ($N = 62$) met full diagnostic criteria for PTSD, 23% met criteria for major depression, and 45% met criteria for any diagnosis (including PTSD, major depression, generalized anxiety disorder, panic disorder, alcohol abuse/dependence, or drug abuse/dependence assessed in this study; North et al., 1999). When PTSD was present, 63% of the time a comorbid post-disaster psychiatric disorder was also diagnosed. The comorbid PTSD was associated with significantly greater evidence of problems functioning compared with PTSD occurring solo.

Most survivors (96%) acknowledged having had at least one PTSD symptom at baseline, and 79% and 82% respectively met symptom group B and D criteria. Therefore, the large majority of the sample was symptomatic of PTSD, with Group B (intrusion) and D (hyperarousal) symptoms apparently representing normative responses, because most of these people did not have PTSD.

Meeting criteria for PTSD symptom group C (avoidance and numbing) significantly predicted meeting full PTSD criteria. Individuals reporting three or more group C symptoms had a 94% chance of meeting full PTSD criteria. In the absence of meeting group C criteria, meeting groups B and D was not associated with a diagnosis of PTSD. Meeting group C criteria was also associated with post-disaster psychiatric comorbidity, psychiatric premorbidity, seeking treatment, taking psychotropic medication for post-disaster symptoms, coping with the bombing by drinking alcohol, and reported problems functioning (North et al., 1999). The prediction of PTSD by the Group C avoidance and numbing criteria is an important advance over previous observations that other early post-disaster symptoms also predict PTSD because the symptoms have been established to be new after the event if the diagnostic criteria are properly assessed, and also because analysis showed that the relationship between Group C and PTSD is specific and not shared by Group B and D criteria. Findings from other studies that early post-disaster dissociative symptoms and panic attacks show associations with later PTSD may be confounded by pre-existing psychopathology or may be nonspecific predictors related to individual symptom reporting style.

The Oklahoma City bombing study follow-up assessment identified 12 additional PTSD cases not diagnosed at baseline, providing a cumulative post-bombing PTSD prevalence rate of 41%. Most of these 12 "new" cases had lacked one or two C symptoms at baseline that they reported at follow-up, thus crossing the diagnostic threshold and representing cases diagnosable only at follow-up. However, the PTSD in all of these 12 cases had begun before six months post-bombing, categorizing them as subthreshold rather than delayed onset cases by *DSM-IV* (American Psychiatric Association, 1994) definition. All identified cases of PTSD had persisted for more than three months, classifying them by *DSM-IV* definition as chronic cases. Therefore, the combined database yielded no cases of PTSD that could be characterized as delayed in onset or as acute in terms of duration.

At follow-up, 31% of the sample was assessed to have current PTSD (in the last month). These numbers might seem to suggest that there was virtually no recovery from PTSD, but six of the 56 individuals with PTSD at any time since the bombing (11%) were in remission from the disorder at follow-up.

## METHODOLOGICAL CONSIDERATIONS

### Psychiatric Assessment

An extensive literature on mental health effects of disasters and terrorism brings to light several pertinent issues related to diagnostic assessment. One of the most critical of these is whether psychiatric *disorders* or *symptoms* are measured. Because after disasters most people experience some PTSD symptoms, the significance of these symptoms loses predictive value. In Oklahoma City, where most survivors met full symptom criteria for intrusion and hyperarousal, the value of intrusion and hyperarousal symptoms for differentiating outcomes is further reduced. Because most people exposed to disasters–even those with direct exposure to very severe disasters such as the Oklahoma City bombing–do not become psychiatrically ill, the word "symptoms" to describe the general psychiatric aftereffects of disasters on populations unnecessarily pathologizes this experience. If there is no disease then one cannot technically have symptoms, which imply disease. More neutral terms for nondiagnostic psychological aftereffects of such extreme events might include "experiences," "reactions," or "responses."

In comparing disaster studies, it is important to consider consistency in assessment of psychopathology. Symptom prevalence, for example, cannot meaningfully be compared to diagnostic prevalence. An illustrative example is the observation that the Oklahoma City bombing study found no new cases of substance use disorders after the disaster, while studies of the terrorist attacks in New York City described significant post-9/11 increases in consumption of alcohol, drugs, and cigarettes (Vlahov et al., 2002). The findings of these studies do not necessarily conflict. Together they suggest that while short-term use of substances may increase after disasters, the increase may not translate into new cases of substance use disorders over subsequent months.

A similar but less obvious source of noncomparability of mental health outcomes in disaster studies is incomplete assessment of the diagnostic criteria for PTSD. Because validity of PTSD assessment by *DSM* criteria depends on adherence to the criteria, apparent disparities in PTSD prevalence between studies may reflect inconsistency of diagnostic assessment more than actual differences in affected populations.

The group B (intrusion) symptoms, for example, must be tied to the context of the traumatic event to be counted toward the diagnosis of PTSD. Because nightmares are a common experience in the general population, even among people who have not experienced a recent traumatic event, failure to tie the content of the nightmares specifically to the event of interest will generate spurious symptoms. Similarly, symptoms in the B and D groups must be *new* after the event to qualify toward the diagnosis of PTSD. Sleep difficulties are endemic and fairly prevalent in the general population; therefore, sleep disturbance cannot be counted toward a diagnosis of PTSD among lifetime poor sleepers even if their sleep difficulties include the post-disaster period. Further, the symptoms must endure for at least a month before a diagnosis of PTSD can be entertained. This is because many people develop multiple post-disaster symptoms that diminish over time rather than proliferating into the full PTSD syndrome. (The diagnosis of Acute Stress Disorder was developed to permit diagnosis during the first month before PTSD may be invoked, but the validity of this diagnosis is not established.) Additionally, the symptoms must result in significant distress (such as taking the person to the doctor) or report of difficulty functioning (such as inability to work).

Many popular clinical and research tools for PTSD assessment, especially self-report questionnaires, fail to address many or all of the above concerns. Some instruments merely inquire about symptoms experienced in the last two weeks and generate diagnoses based on symptom counts or scales constructed from symptom frequency or severity. Each diagnostic criterion of PTSD unaddressed by an instrument of assessment further inflates estimated PTSD prevalence. Structured diagnostic interviews that painstakingly assess all PTSD criteria yield considerably lower rates of PTSD compared to self-report questionnaires (Rubonis & Bickman, 1991). The reason behind their infrequent use, however, is the labor-intensive, resource-draining nature of structured diagnostic assessment that tends to be prohibitive in most studies.

Not only is post-disaster diagnosis important, but documentation of pre-disaster diagnosis is also of considerable interest. For example, a study of rescue and recovery workers involved in the Oklahoma City bombing found a 24% prevalence of alcohol abuse or dependence afterward, but almost all of the cases were pre-existing (North et al., 2002). New cases of alcohol use disorders after traumatic events would represent quite a different concept from those predating the event in terms of both choosing treatment and also in prognosticating mental health outcomes.

### Sampling

The Oklahoma City bombing sample represents a directly exposed group, in which one might expect to find the highest rates of psychopathology of any exposure group. Less directly exposed groups might be expected to show milder psychiatric effects. For example, the 34% prevalence of PTSD after the bombing in Oklahoma City was quite a bit higher than the 8% (Galea et al., 2002) to 11% (Schlenger et al., 2002) rates reported after the September 11th World Trade Center attacks among the residential population of Manhattan. The difference in the results can be traced to sampling differences: the highly exposed sample in Oklahoma City (all in the direct path of the bomb blast and 87% injured) compared to the population of Manhattan not sampled based on exposure to the attacks (largely indirectly exposed people at various distances, often miles, from Ground Zero at the time of the attacks).

## *Analysis of Longitudinal Data*

Follow-up data from the Oklahoma City bombing study support other disaster literature in finding that multiple assessments over time increase the yield of identified PTSD cases. Not previously reported, however, is the finding that detection of psychiatric illness and recovery from it requires comparison of individual data over time rather than examination of summary rates of diagnoses or symptoms. In Oklahoma City, the presentation of baseline and follow-up PTSD data revealed similar rates that masked activity embedded in the data. Over time, some people recovered from PTSD, but they were obscured in the summary statistics by similar numbers of people with worsening illness.

## *CONCLUSIONS*

The Oklahoma City bombing study (North et al., 1999) provided useful information for clinicians about mental health effects of terrorism among highly exposed populations in the first six months after the event. Longitudinal data provided additional relevant information and within-person analysis of the data revealed individual changes over time that were masked by presentation of summary statistics alone. The yield of identified PTSD cases increased with a second assessment, and a more complete and optimistic picture of the course of PTSD emerged by examination of remission rates across time. Review of additional methodological issues in this report has clarified the importance of diagnostic assessment compared to symptom measurement, adherence to established criteria in estimating the prevalence of psychiatric disorders, and orientation of mental health outcomes to the type of disaster exposure of the sample.

Potential clinical implications of the Oklahoma City bombing study of survivors of the direct bomb blast are the following: (1) people are highly resilient, given that two-thirds of the directly exposed survivors of this severe disaster did not develop PTSD; (2) post-disaster diagnostic assessment should not stop with the diagnosis of PTSD, as the disorder is more often comorbid with another psychiatric disorder than not, with the presence of cormorbidity identifying the most distressed and functionally impaired cases; (3) because PTSD starts early, interventions may begin early with screening the affected population for avoidance and numbing symptoms that are highly indicative of the disorder (a finding that awaits replication in prospective studies); and (4) because PTSD tends toward chronicity, mental health interventions are needed over the long haul for persistent cases (not the same as delayed-onset PTSD which is not characteristic after disasters).

## REFERENCES

Abenhaim, L. (1992). Study of civilian victims of terrorist attacks (France 1982-1987). *Journal of Clinical Epidemiology, 45*, 103-109.

American Psychiatric Association. (1994). *Diagnostic and statistical manual of mental disorders, 4th ed.* Washington, DC: Author.

Amir, M., Weil, G., Kaplan, Z., Tocker, T., & Witztum, E. (1998). Debriefing with brief group psychotherapy in a homogenous group of non-injured victims of a terrorist attack: A prospective study. *Acta Psychiatrica Scandinavica, 98*, 237-242.

Curran, P.S., Bell, P., Murray, A., Loughrey, G., Roddy, R., & Rocke, L.G. (1990). Psychological consequences of the Enniskillen bombing. *British Journal of Psychiatry, 156*, 479-482.

Epstein, R., Fullerton, C., & Ursano, R. (1998). Posttraumatic stress disorder following an air disaster: A prospective study. *American Journal of Psychiatry, 155*, 934-938.

Galea, S., Ahern, J., Resnick, H., Kilpatrick, D., Bucuvalis, M., Gold, J., & Vlahov, D. (2002). Psychological sequelae of the September 11 terrorist attacks in New York City. *New England Journal of Medicine, 346*, 982-987.

Grace, M.C., Green, B.L., Lindy, J.L., & Leonard, A.C. (1993). The Buffalo Creek Disaster: A 14-year follow-up. In J.P. Wilson & B. Raphael (Eds.), *International handbook of traumatic stress syndromes* (pp. 441-449). New York: Plenum Press.

Groenjian, A.K., Steinberg, A.M., Najarian, L.M., Fairbanks, L.A., Tashjian, M., & Pynoos, R.S. (2000). Prospective study of posttraumatic stress, anxiety, and depressive reactions after earthquake and political violence. *American Journal of Psychiatry, 157*, 911-916.

Johnson, S.D., North, C.S., & Smith, E.M. (2002). Psychiatric disorders among victims of a courthouse shooting spree: A three-year follow-up study. *Community Mental Health Journal, 38*, 181-194.

McFarlane, A. (1988). The longitudinal course of posttraumatic morbidity: The range of outcomes and their predictors. *Journal of Nervous and Mental Disease, 176*, 30-39.

North, C.S., McCutcheon, V., Spitznagel, E.L., & Smith, E.M. (2002). Three-year follow-up of survivors of a mass shooting episode. *Journal of Urban Health, 79*, 383-391.

North, C.S., Nixon, S.J., Shariat, S., Mallonee, S., McMillen, J.C., Spitznagel, E.L., & Smith, E.M. (1999). Psychiatric disorders among survivors of the Oklahoma City bombing. *Journal of the American Medical Association, 282*, 755-762.

North, C.S., Smith, E.M., & Spitznagel, E.L. (1997). One-year follow-up of survivors of a mass shooting. *American Journal of Psychiatry, 154*, 1696-1702.

North, C.S., Tivis, L., McMillen, J.C., Pfefferbaum, B., Spitznagel, E.L., Cox, J., Nixon, S., Bunch, K.P., & Smith, E.M. (2002). Psychiatric disorders in rescue workers after the Oklahoma City bombing. *American Journal of Psychiatry, 159*, 857-859.

Rubonis, A.V., & Bickman, L. (1991). Psychological impairment in the wake of disaster: The disaster-psychopathology relationship. *Psychological Bulletin, 109*, 384-399.

Schlenger, W.E., Caddell, J.M., Ebert, L., Jordan, B.K., Rourke, K.M., Wilson, D., Thalji, L., Dennis, J.M., Fairbank, J.A., & Kulka, R.A. (2002). Psychological reactions to terrorist attacks: Findings from the National Study of Americans' Reactions to September 11. *Journal of the American Medical Association, 288*, 581-588.

Shalev, A.Y. (1992). Posttraumatic stress disorder among injured survivors of a terrorist attack: Predictive value of early intrusion and avoidance symptoms. *Journal of Nervous and Mental Disease, 180*, 505-509.

Steinglass, P., & Gerrity, E. (1990). Natural disasters and posttraumatic stress disorder: Short-term vs. long-term recovery in two disaster-affected communities. *Journal of Applied Social Psychology, 20*, 1746-1765.

Ursano, R.J., Fullerton, C.S., Kao, T., & Bhartiya, V. R. (1995). Longitudinal assessment of posttraumatic stress disorder and depression after exposure to traumatic death. *Journal of Nervous and Mental Disease, 183*, 36-42.

Vlahov, D., Galea, S., Resnick, H., Ahern, J., Boscarino, J.A., Bucavalas, M., Gold, J., & Kilpatrick, D. (2002). Increased use of cigarettes, alcohol, and marijuana among Manhattan, New York, residents after the September 11th terrorist attacks. *American Journal of Epidemiology, 155*, 988-996.

Wang, X., Gao, L., Shinfuku, N., Zhang, H., Zhao, C., & Shen, Y. (2000). Longitudinal study of earthquake-related PTSD in a randomly selected community sample in north China. *American Journal of Psychiatry, 157*, 1260-1266.

Weisaeth, L. (1985). Post-traumatic stress disorder after an industrial disaster. In P. Pichot, P. Berner, R. Wolf, & K. Thau (Eds.), *Psychiatry–The state of the art* (pp. 299-307). New York: Plenum Press.

# Risk Factors for Acute Stress Disorder in Children with Burns

Glenn Saxe, MD
Frederick Stoddard, MD
Neharika Chawla, MA
Carlos G. Lopez, MD
Erin Hall, MA
Robert Sheridan, MD
Daniel King, PhD
Lynda King, PhD

**SUMMARY.** The purpose of this study was to (1) estimate the prevalence of acute stress disorder (ASD) in a sample of burned children, and (2) determine risk factors for ASD in these children. Seventy-two chil-

Glenn Saxe, Neharika Chawla, Carlos G. Lopez, Erin Hall, Daniel King, and Lynda King are affiliated with the Department of Child and Adolescent Psychiatry, Boston Medical Center, Boston University School of Medicine, Boston, MA, and the National Child Traumatic Stress Network. Daniel King and Lynda King are also affiliated with the Veterans Administration New England Healthcare System. Frederick Stoddard and Robert Sheridan are affiliated with the Department of Psychiatry, Shriners Burns Hospital and Harvard Medical School, Boston, MA.

Address correspondence to: Glenn Saxe, MD, Department of Child and Adolescent Psychiatry, Dowling 1 North, One Boston Medical Center Place, Boston, MA 02118 (E-mail: glenn.saxe@bmc.org).

The research described in this paper was supported by NIMH grant R01 MH57370 and SAMHSA grant U79 SM54305 (Dr. Saxe).

[Haworth co-indexing entry note]: "Risk Factors for Acute Stress Disorder in Children with Burns." Saxe, Glenn et al. Co-published simultaneously in *Journal of Trauma & Dissociation* (The Haworth Medical Press, an imprint of The Haworth Press, Inc.) Vol. 6, No. 2, 2005, pp. 37-49; and: *Acute Reactions to Trauma and Psychotherapy: A Multidisciplinary and International Perspective* (ed: Etzel Cardeña, and Kristin Croyle) The Haworth Medical Press, an imprint of The Haworth Press, Inc., 2005, pp. 37-49. Single or multiple copies of this article are available for a fee from The Haworth Document Delivery Service [1-800-HAWORTH, 9:00 a.m. - 5:00 p.m. (EST). E-mail address: docdelivery@haworthpress.com].

dren were assessed for acute stress disorder approximately 10 days after being hospitalized for a burn. Variables hypothesized to predict ASD symptoms (i.e., size of the burn, prior behavioral symptoms, body image, parents' symptoms, heart rate) were also assessed. Based on a diagnosis derived from the ASD module of the Diagnostic Interview for Children and Adolescents (DICA), 31% of children met criteria for ASD. Path analyses revealed that the variables of heart rate, body image, and parents' acute stress symptoms were directly related to the development of ASD symptoms and accounted for 41% of its variance. These variables also mediated the relationship between the size of the burn and ASD symptoms. ASD is found in almost one third of children hospitalized for a burn. A high resting heart rate, lowered body image, and parent's acute stress symptoms were found to be significant risk factors for ASD symptoms. *[Article copies available for a fee from The Haworth Document Delivery Service: 1-800-HAWORTH. E-mail address: <docdelivery@ haworthpress.com> Website: <http://www.HaworthPress.com> © 2005 by The Haworth Press, Inc. All rights reserved.]*

**KEYWORDS.** Acute stress disorder, ASD, burns, children

Of the two million individuals who suffer from burn injuries in the United States each year, approximately half are children (American Burn Association, 1984; Silverstein & Lack, 1987). Fire and burn injuries are the third leading cause of death in children in the United States (Guyer & Gallager, 1985). Estimates from an economic analysis suggest that in the United States in 1985 alone, pediatric burns resulted in a loss of more than 101,000 life years with a societal cost of more than 3.5 billion dollars (McLoughlin & McGuire, 1990).

The burn itself is almost always unexpected and usually very painful for children. Shortly after the burn, children frequently find themselves on an intensive care unit where they may undergo extensive surgery. The hospitalization involves separation of children from their families, who themselves are occasionally injured or killed. Recovery in the hospital usually involves painful dressing changes, and often children must adjust to permanent changes in their body's appearance and function. The traumatic nature of burn injuries in children is compounded by the fact that 6-20% are related to child abuse or neglect (Caniano, Beaver & Bowles, 1986; Purdue, Hunt & Prescott, 1988; Renze & Sherman, 1993).

Children hospitalized with an acute burn frequently develop severe psychological reactions such as nightmares, flashbacks, behavioral regressions, and posttraumatic play (Kravitz et al., 1993; Stoddard, 1985; Stoddard, Murphy, Rizzone, unpublished manuscript; Stoddard, Norman, Murphy & Beardslee, 1989; Tarnowski & Rasnake, 1994). The psychological intensity of burn trauma, and particularly the relentless stress of hospital treatment for a burn, has been compared to "inescapable shock" or "learned helplessness" (Kavanaugh et al., 1991) both of which have been described as models of PTSD (Charney, Deutch, Krystal, Southwick, & Davis, 1993; van der Kolk, 1994). Between 25% and 33% of burn-injured children eventually develop PTSD and over fifty percent display some posttraumatic symptoms (Stoddard, 1985; Stoddard et al., 1989). Children with burns also develop mood, anxiety, sleep, conduct, elimination, learning, and attentional problems (Kravitz et al., 1993; Stoddard, 1985; Stoddard et al., unpublished manuscript; Stoddard et al., 1989; Tarnowski & Rasnake, 1994).

Symptoms of hyperarousal/anxiety, and dissociation are the main features of the acute response to trauma. This response was formally recognized in the *Diagnostic and Statistical Manual of Mental Disorders-IV* (*DSM IV*; APA, 1994) with addition of Acute Stress Disorder (ASD). ASD describes the psychopathological response in the immediate aftermath of a traumatic event that occurs up until one month following the trauma. Daviss, Racusin, Fleischer, Mooney, Ford, and McHugo (2000) and Koplin Winston et al. (2002) have reported a broad range of ASD symptoms in separate cohorts of injured children.

Numerous studies have documented the increased prevalence of PTSD in those initially diagnosed with ASD. For example, Harvey and Bryant (2000) diagnosed PTSD in 78% of victims of motor vehicle accidents six months following the accident. Brewin, Andrews, Rose, and Kirk (1999) reported that a diagnosis of ASD predicted PTSD in 83% of assault victims. Bryant, Harvey, Guthrie, and Moulds (2000), in an interesting study that included ASD and psychophysiological parameters, found that ASD and a high resting heart rate predicted PTSD in motor vehicle accident victims with 88% sensitivity and 85% specificity. Holeva and colleagues reported that motor vehicle accident victims with ASD were 20 times more likely to receive a diagnosis of PTSD (Holeva, Tarrier & Wells, 2001). Thus it is clear that ASD is an important early response to traumatic events and is related to PTSD.

Although a burn and the subsequent hospitalization for burn care are unquestionably traumatic events, there have been few studies of children in the acute aftermath of a burn and, to our knowledge, no studies of ASD in the acute aftermath of a burn amongst children. In fact there are few studies of the prevalence and risk factors for ASD among any population of traumatized children. ASD has never been studied among children with burns. The goal of this study is to estimate the prevalence of ASD among children hospitalized with a burn injury and to determine risk factors for the development of ASD.

## METHODS

### Participants

The participants were a sample of children admitted to Shriners Burns Hospital in Boston, for an acute burn. All children aged 7 to 17 years were eligible to participate unless they or their parents did not speak sufficient English to complete the study instruments. Our sample consisted of 72 children. The mean age of these children was 11.20 years ($SD = 3.51$); 24 were girls and 48 were boys. The average length of stay was 25 days ($SD = 22.77$). Mean body surface area burned was 17.58% (range 1-85%). The participants completed an interview administered by a research assistant as soon as they were medically stable (e.g., they did not have a delirium, an active infection, and were not receiving mechanical ventilation, etc.). Medical stability was determined by the attending surgeon at Shriners Burns Hospital. Children were interviewed an average of 10 days after admission (range 2-26 days).

## PROCEDURES

One or more parents of a prospective child participant were approached by one of the investigators, and the nature of the study was explained. Once written informed consent had been obtained from the parent, and written informed assent was obtained from the child, the initial interview was completed. Children were interviewed using the ASD module of the Diagnostic Interview for Children and Adolescents-*DSM IV* (DICA; Reich, 2000). Children also completed the Piers-Harris Self Concept Scale (PHSCS; Piers, 1984) as part of a larger assessment battery. Additionally, the child's parent completed the Child Stress Disorders Checklist to measure their child's ASD symptoms and The Coddington Life Events Scale (LES; Coddington, 1972; Holmes & Rahe, 1967) about the child's exposure to stressful life events from before the burn. The parent also completed the Stanford Acute Stress Reaction Questionnaire (SASRQ; Cardeña, Koopman, Classen, Waelde, & Spiegel, 2000) about their own symptoms of ASD. The child's nurse also completed the Child Stress Disorders Checklist (CSDC; Saxe et al., 2003) in order to assess the child's acute stress reactions. A chart review was conducted to gather information about the child's heart rate throughout the hospital stay. Heart rate was recorded by the child's nurse 4-12 times per day during the hospitalization. Each participant was assigned a numerical identification code in order to ensure participant anonymity.

## Measures

The Diagnostic Interview for Children and Adolescents (DICA; Reich, 2000) is a broad-based semi-structured interview schedule that includes a PTSD module, and has been widely used in clinical and non-clinical populations. It has been employed in a number of different samples of traumatized children including victims of earthquakes and burns, refugees, and abused children. As found with many diagnostic interviews of children, there is a questionable degree of reliability between responses derived from parents and children on this instrument, but a high degree of inter-rater reliability ($k = .76$).

Our group added a number of items to the PTSD module of the DICA in order to derive a diagnosis of ASD. The diagnosis of ASD was derived from the PTSD module of the DICA, using items that assessed each of the *DSM IV* criteria for ASD. The diagnostic criteria were altered by increasing the required number of dissociative symptoms (criterion B) to three and reducing the number of required symptoms for avoidance (criterion D) and increased arousal (criterion E). Internal consistency reliability was found to be .91. In a sample of 17 children, we found perfect inter-rater agreement at the diagnostic level ($k = 1.00$). In order to determine validity we correlated number of ASD symptoms to other measures of acute stress, PTSD symptomatology and trauma severity. The number of symptoms was significantly correlated to scores on the CSDC, as reported by parents ($r = .30$, $p < .05$), and to scores on the Child PTSD Reaction Index (Nader, 1990; Nader, Pynoos, & Fairbanks, 1996; $r = .74$, $p < .01$). As the DICA ASD module is designed as a diagnostic assessment, it was used in this study to estimate the prevalence of ASD in burned children.

The Child Stress Disorders Checklist (Saxe et al., 2003) is a 36-item observer-report instrument that measures acute stress and posttraumatic stress symptoms in children. It is the first instrument designed to be an appropriate measure of the symptoms of ASD in children, when administered within one month of the trauma, and it includes items that measure acute dissociation. The CSDC matches the response format of the CBCL. Each symptom is rated on a 3-point scale (0 = "not true"; 1 = "somewhat true"; 2 = "very true"). The CSDC was found to be internally consistent in a sample of 103 children who had either been burned, been in a traffic crash, or experienced abuse (*alpha* = .91). Test retest reliability in this sample of burned children was .84. Scores on the CSDC were also found to be moderately correlated to well established measures of trauma-related symptomatology. The scores from the nurses' report were also significantly correlated to percentage of body surface area burned, an index of trauma severity, with $r = .43$ ($p < .01$). As the CSRC is designed to be a continuous scale of ASD symptoms it was our main dependent variable in the path analytic component of this study.

The Coddington Life Events Scale (LES; Coddington, 1972; Holmes & Rahe, 1967) identifies life events experienced by the participant and significant others in the past year. Items included in the measure were based on earlier instruments applied to the field of child psychiatry and relevant to the child and adolescent age groups. The Coddington scales have been developed and utilized across multiple socioeconomic and ethnic groups. Examples of items are: (1) the death of a parent, (2) birth of a brother or sister, (3) failing a grade in school, (4) appearance in juvenile court, (5) illness in the family, and (6) loss of a parent's job.

The Piers-Harris Children's Self Concept Scale (PHSCS; Piers, 1984) is an 80-item self-report measure that requires the child to evaluate his or her own behavior and attributes. A high score on this scale reflects a positive self-evaluation and a low score reflects a negative self-evaluation. This instrument has six different "cluster scales": behavior, intellectual and school status, physical appearance and attributes, anxiety, popularity, and happiness and satisfaction. Each of these scales measures self-concept or self-esteem derived from its respective source. Test-retest reliability coefficients on this scale have ranged from .42 to .96. Internal consistency estimates of the total score range from .88 to .93. This instrument also appears to have sufficient convergent and discriminant validity.

The Stanford Acute Stress Reaction Questionnaire (SASRQ; Cardeña et al., 2000) is a 30-item questionnaire designed to evaluate acute stress in accordance with the *DSM-IV* criteria for Acute Stress Disorder (ASD). The items on the questionnaire assess dissociation, reexperiencing, avoidance, anxiety, hyperarousal, and impairment in functioning. Across varied samples and studies, the scale has demonstrated very good reliability (alpha range: .87-.95) and strong construct, predictive, discriminant, and convergent validity.

The mean pulse rate was calculated by our research nurse in a review of the vital signs sheets of the hospital record. All children had their vital signs (pulse rate, blood pressure) assessed 4-12 times per day by the child's clinical nurse and noted in the "vital signs" sheets of the medical record. The value of mean pulse rate was derived through calculating the mean of all these observations of the child's pulse rate throughout their hospital stay.

## Statistical Analyses

*Prevalence of ASD.* Based on the child's appraisal of acute stress items on the DICA, we specified the percentage of our sample that met criterion for each ASD symptom group. Based on whether they met full criteria or not, participants were classified as having ASD or no ASD.

*Risk factors for ASD.* We used a path analytic strategy to examine the results, similar to that used by Shalev, Peri, Canetti, and Schreiber (1996) in another prospective study of acutely traumatized individuals. As this strategy follows a prospective longitudinal methodology, the directionality of many of the paths are constrained by the time that the variables were assessed. Accordingly, we divided variables into (1) ASD symptoms (our main dependent variable), (2) peri-traumatic variables (variables assessed shortly after the trauma), (3) trauma exposure variable (percentage of body surface area burned), and (4) pre-trauma variables (variables about the child/family from before the trauma). A series of hierarchically-nested, ordinary least squares multiple regression analyses were used in order to estimate direct and indirect effects among variables. The first step was to predict the dependent variable (ASD symptoms). In order to constrain the number of paths in this model, we deleted paths whose bivariate relationships with ASD were less than 0.20. Of the remaining variables, we began to choose combinations of variables that accounted for a high percentage of the variance of PTSD symptoms (high $R^2$), guided by our theoretical understanding of ASD. Once these variables were chosen we began to build a model of mediation. That is to say, we examined the series of variables "upstream" from ASD guided by our theoretical model and constrained by bivariate relationships that were stronger than 0.20. As described above, we were further constrained by temporal relationships. The direction of relationships chosen must make temporal sense (e.g., ASD symptoms could not lead to pre-traumatic life stress; peri-traumatic pulse rate

FIGURE 1. Path analytic model of the development of ASD. Betas for each pathway are depicted above the arrows.

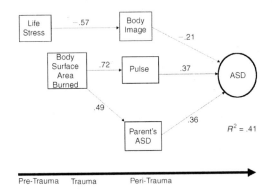

could not lead to the size of the burn). In this way a network of relationships between variables was chosen, as illustrated in Figure 1 that, as discussed below, adds important understanding to the development of ASD.

*Approach to missing data.* Problems related to missing data can reduce the number of participants for a particular analysis to a less than optimal level. We employed the statistical package "M-plus 2.1" (Muthen & Muthen, 1998) full information maximum likelihood estimator to retain complete sample size for each analysis. M-plus is preferred since it is able to use the full information maximum likelihood procedure in concert with the Satorra-Bentler correction for non-normal data (see the work of McArdle and Cattell (1994), and Graham, Hofer, Donaldson, MacKinnon, and Schafer (1997) for discussion of the advantages of imputation over more traditional listwise and pairwise deletion procedures).

## RESULTS

### Prevalence of ASD

In our sample of 72 children, 87% met ASD criterion A (traumatic event), 44% met criterion B (dissociation), 79% met criterion C (reexperiencing), 44% met criterion D (avoidance) and 72% met criterion E (hyperarousal). Within criterion B; 43% displayed one or more symptoms of numbing, 48% displayed reduced awareness of surroundings, 61% demonstrated derealization, 45% displayed depersonalization, and 37% displayed dissociative amnesia. Thirty-one percent of our sample of children met full criteria for ASD within two weeks following the burn. To meet criterion A, subjects must have endorsed at least one A2 (immediate response) item.

### Risk Factors for ASD

According to the aforementioned protocol, we chose three variables (parent's ASD symptoms, body image, and pulse rate) that accounted for 41% of the variance of PTSD ($R^2 = .41$). We then built a model of mediation using body surface area burned and life stress from before the burn. Figure 1 displays the results of the model with standardized regression coefficients (*betas*) given for each path. As can be seen, the size of the burn (i.e., Body Surface Area Burned) was only related to ASD via its influence on pulse rate and parent's ASD symptoms, respectively. Life stresses from before the burn also influenced the development of ASD but via its impact on the child's body image. The model yielded strong fit indices, using the Chi Square ($\chi^2 = 9.74$, $df = 8$, $p = .28$), the Comparative Fit Index ($CFI = .97$) and the Root Mean Square Error of Approximation ($RMSEA = .056$).

### DISCUSSION

Almost a third of the participants met *DSM-IV* criteria for ASD. Our path analysis model of the development of ASD yielded three variables that together accounted for 41% of the variance of ASD. These variables were (1) the parent's symptoms of ASD (measured by the Stanford Acute Stress Reaction Questionnaire), (2) the child's mean pulse rate (measured numerous times during his or her hospitalization), and (3) the child's body image (measured with the Piers Harris Self Concept Scale). The magnitude of the trauma (defined as the percentage of body surface area burned) did not affect ASD directly but only via its influence on the parent's symptoms, and the child's mean pulse rate. Similarly, life stress before the burn only influenced ASD via its effect on the child's body image.

There is a growing literature on the relationship between heart rate and traumatic stress. Shalev et al. (1998) has reported close associations between heart rate and the development of PTSD. Heart rate is an index of noradrenergic activity, which has strong associations with PTSD (Kosten, Mason, Giller, Ostroff, & Harkness, 1987; Perry, Giller, & Southwick, 1987; Southwick et al., 1993). Pitman (1989) has speculated that the hyperadrenergic state occurring in the wake of a traumatic event is responsible for the over-consolidation of traumatic memory in those who develop traumatic stress responses. This over-consolidation of the traumatic memory then becomes manifest in the intrusive memories and re-experiencing of traumatic stress. The recall of the traumatic event leads to the re-release of catecholamines and stress hormones that further enhance the traumatic memory. Our finding on the association between heart rate and ASD is consistent with this literature and has implications for acute intervention. Pitman (1989) and Saxe et al. (2001) have proposed the use of agents that block the noradrenergic system in acutely traumatized individuals as possible preventative agents for PTSD.

Our data on parents' acute stress symptoms predicting children's symptoms is important and suggests that parents who are overwhelmed with their own symptoms (and who may be triggered by their child) may have diminished capacity to help their child while they are recovering following a burn. Alternatively the relationship between parent and child PTSD may indicate shared biologic or genetic vulnerability to traumatic stress. Such findings suggest that parents must be carefully assessed and offered treatment if they are developing ASD.

Children with burns often have extensive damage to the appearance and functioning of their bodies. The maintenance of a positive body image following a burn has been suggested as an important protective factor (Orr, Reznikoff, & Smith, 1989; Stoddard, 1982). Our finding that a positive body image is inversely related to ASD symptoms is consistent with this notion and suggests that interventions that help children enhance body image may have great value in the care of burned children.

In summary, almost a third of children hospitalized for a burn injury met DSM IV criteria for ASD. Risk factors for ASD symptoms included the parent's level of ASD, the child's pulse rate, and the child's body image. The size of the burn was only indirectly related to the development of ASD.

# REFERENCES

American Burn Association. (1984). Guidelines for service standards and severity classification in the treatment of burn injuries. *Bulletin of the American College of Surgeons, 69,* 24-28.

American Psychiatric Association. (1994). *Diagnostic and statistical manual, 4th ed.* Washington, DC: Author.

Brewin, C.R. Andrews, B., Rose, S., & Kirk, M. (1999). Acute stress disorder and posttraumatic stress disorder in victims of violent crime. *American Journal of Psychiatry, 156,* 360-365.

Bryant, R.A., Harvey, A.G., Guthrie, R., & Moulds, M. (2000). A prospective study of acute psychophysiological arousal, acute stress disorder, and posttraumatic stress disorder. *Journal of Abnormal Psychology, 109,* 341-344.

Caniano, D.A., Beaver, B.L., & Bowles, E.T. (1986). Child abuse: An update on surgical management of 256 cases. *Annals of Surgery, 203,* 219-224.

Cardeña, E., Koopman, C., Classen, C., Waelde, L.C., & Spiegel, D. (2000). Psychometric properties of the Stanford Acute Stress Reaction Questionnaire (SASRQ): A valid and reliable measure of acute stress. *Journal of Traumatic Stress, 13,* 719-734.

Charney, D.C., Deutch, A.Y., Krystal, J.H., Southwick, & Davis, M. (1993). Psychobiological mechanisms of posttraumatic stress disorder. *Archives of General Psychiatry, 50,* 294-305.

Coddington, R.D. (1972). The significance of life events as etiological factors in the diseases of children: II. A study of a normal population. *Journal of Psychosomatic Research, 16,* 205-213.

Daviss, W.B., Racusin, R., Fleischer, A., Mooney, D., Ford, J.D., & McHugo, G.J. (2000). Acute stress disorder symptomatology during hospitalization for pediatric injury. *Journal of the American Academy of Child and Adolescent Psychiatry, 39,* 569-75.

Graham, J.W., Hofer, S.M., Donaldson, S.I., MacKinnon, D.P., & Schafer, J.L. (1997). Analysis with missing data in prevention research. In K.J. Bryant, M. Windle, & S. G. West (Eds.), *The science of prevention: Methodological advances from alcohol and substance abuse research* (pp. 325-366). Washington, DC: American Psychological Association.

Guyer, B., & Gallagher, S.S. (1985). An approach to the epidemiology of childhood injuries. *Pediatric Clinics of North America, 32,* 5-15.

Harvey, A.G., & Bryant, R.A. (2000). Two-year prospective evaluation of the relationship between acute stress disorder and posttraumatic stress disorder following mild traumatic brain injury. *American Journal of Psychiatry, 157,* 626-628.

Holeva, V., Tarrier, N., & Wells, A. (2001). Prevalence and predictors of acute stress disorder and PTSD following road traffic accidents: Thought control strategies and social support. *Behaviour Therapy, 32,* 65-83.

Holmes, T.H., & Rahe, R.H. (1967). The social readjustment rating scale. *Journal of Psychosomatic Research, 11,* 213-218.

Kavanagh, C.K., Lasoff, E., Eide, Y, Freeman, R., McEttrick, M., Dar, R., Helgerson, R., Remensnyder, J. & Kalin, N. (1991). Learned helplessness and the pediatric burn patient: Dressing change behavior and serum cortisol and beta-endorphin. In L.A. Barness, A. Bongiovanni, G. Morrow, F.A. Oski, & A.M., Rudolf (Eds.), *Advances in pediatrics* (vol. 38, pp. 335-362). Chicago: Year Book.

Kosten, T.R., Mason, J.W., Giller, E.L., Ostroff, R.B., & Harkness, L. (1987). Sustained urinary norepinepherine and epinepherine elevation in PTSD. *Psychoneuroendocrinology, 12,* 13-20.

Kravitz, M., McCoy, B.J.M., Tomkins, D.M., Daly W., Mulligan J., McCauley, R.L., Robson, M.C., & Herndon, D.N. (1993). Sleep disorders in children after burn injury. *Journal of Burn Care Rehabilitation, 14,* 83-90.

McArdle, J.J., & Cattell, R.B. (1994). Structural equation models of factorial invariance in parallel proportional profiles and oblique cofactor problems. *Multivariate Behavior Research, 29,* 63-113.

McLoughlin, E., & McGuire, A. (1990). The causes, cost and prevention of childhood burn injuries. *The American Journal of Disorders in Childhood, 144,* 667-671.

Muthen, L.K., & Muthen, B.O. (1998). *M plus Statistical Analysis With Latent Variables: User's Guide.* Los Angeles, CA: Muthen & Muthen.

Nader, K. (1996). Assessing trauma in children. In J. Wilson & T.M. Keane (Eds.), *Assessing psychological trauma and PTSD* (pp. 291-348). New York: Guilford.

Nader, K., Pynoos, R., Fairbanks, J.L. (1990). Children's PTSD reactions one year after a sniper attack on their school. *American Journal of Psychiatry, 147,* 1526-1530.

Orr, D.A., Reznikoff, M., & Smith, G.M. (1989). Body image, self esteem, and depression in burn injured adolescents and young adults. *Journal of Burn Care and Rehabilitation, 10,* 454-461.

Perry, B.D., Giller, E.L., & Southwick, S.M. (1987). Altered plasma alpha-2 adrenergic receptor affinity in PTSD. *American Journal of Psychiatry, 144,* 1511-1512.

Piers, E.V. (1984). *Piers-Harris Children's Self-Concept Scale* (Rev. ed.). Los Angeles: Western Psychological Services.

Pitman, R.K. (1989). Post-traumatic stress disorder, hormones, and memory [editorial]. *Biological Psychiatry, 26,* 221-223.

Purdue, G.F., Hunt, J.L., & Prescott, P.R. (1988). Child burning by abuse: An index of suspicion. *Journal of Trauma, 28,* 221-224.

Renze, B.M., & Sherman, R. (1993). Abusive scald burns in infants and children: A prospective study. *American Surgeon, 58,* 329-334.

Reich, W. (2000). Diagnostic Interview for Children and Adolescents (DICA). *Journal of the American Academy of Child and Adolescent Psychiatry, 39,* 59-66.

Saxe, G., Chawla, N., Stoddard, F., Kassam-Adams, N., Courtney, D., Cunningham, K., Lopez, C., Hall, E., Sheridan, R., King, L. & King, D. (2003). Child Stress Disorders Checklist: A measure of ASD and PTSD in children. *Journal of the American Academy of Child and Adolescent Psychiatry, 42,* 972-978.

Saxe, G., Stoddard, F., Courtney, D., Cunningham, K., Chawla, N., Sheridan, R., King, D., & King, L. (2001). Relationship between acute morphine and the course of PTSD in children with burns. *Journal of the American Academy of Child and Adolescent Psychiatry, 40,* 915-921.

Shalev, A.Y., Peri, T., Canetti, L., & Schreiber, S. (1996). Predictors of PTSD in injured trauma survivors: A prospective study. *American Journal of Psychiatry, 153,* 219-225.

Shalev, A.Y., Sahar, T., Freedman, S., Peri, T., Glick, N., Brandes, D., Orr, S.P., & Pitman, R.K. (1998). A prospective study of heart rate responses following trauma and the subsequent development of posttraumatic stress disorder. *Archives of General Psychiatry, 55,* 553-559.

Silverstein, P., & Lack, B.O. Epidemiology and prevention. In J.A. Boswick (Ed.), *The art and science of burn care* (pp. 11-17). Rockville, MD: Lippincott Williams & Wilkins.

Southwick, S.M., Krystal, J.H., Morgan, A., Johnson, D., Nagy, L.M., Nicolaou, G.R., Heniger, G.R., & Charney, D.S. (1993) Abnormal noradrenergic function in post-traumatic stress disorder. *Archives of General Psychiatry, 50,* 266-274.

Stoddard, F.J. (1982). Body image development in the burned child. *Journal of the American Academy of Child Psychiatry, 21,* 502-507.

Stoddard, F.J. (1985). Care of infants, children and adolescents with burn injuries. In M. Lewis (Ed.), *Child and adolescent psychiatry: A comprehensive textbook* (pp. 1016-1037). Baltimore, MD: Williams and Wilkins.

Stoddard, F.J., Murphy, J.M., Rizzone, L. *PTSD in children after recovery from burns.* Unpublished manuscript.

Stoddard, F.J., Norman, D.K., Murphy, J.M., & Beardslee, W.R. (1989). Psychiatric outcome of burned children. *Journal of the American Academy of Child and Adolescent Psychiatry, 28,* 589-595.

Tarnowski, K.J., & Rasnake, L.K. (1994). Long term psychosocial sequelae. In K.J. Tarnowski (Ed.), *Behavioral aspects of pediatric burns* (pp. 81-118). New York, NY: Plenum Press.

van der Kolk, B.A. (1994). The body keeps the score: Memory and the evolving psychobiology of PTSD. *Harvard Review of Psychiatry, 1,* 253-265.

Winston, F.K., Kassam-Adams, N., Vivarelli-O'Neill, C., Ford, J., Newman, E., Baxt, C., Stafford, P., & Cnaan, A. (2002). Acute Stress Disorder Symptoms in children and their parents after pediatric traffic injury. *Pediatrics, 109,* e90.

# Effects of Traumatic Stress
# on Brain Structure and Function:
# Relevance to Early Responses to Trauma

J. Douglas Bremner, MD

**SUMMARY.** The events of 9/11 and the widening impact of psychological trauma today have raised a higher level of awareness about the potentially deleterious effects of psychological trauma on the individual. One area of interest after 9/11 was the early trauma response and the most effective way to deal with the window of time immediately after traumatization in order to prevent long term psychopathology. Understanding the neurobiology of the acute trauma response may be useful in designing prevention and treatment strategies. Studies in animals and humans have shown that biological stress response systems, including norepinephrine and cortisol, are affected in both the acute and chronic stages of the trauma response. Brain areas involved in memory, including the hippocampus, amygdala, and prefrontal cortex, may be areas of intervention to ameliorate the early trauma response. Due to the difficulty of performing research in this time period, most research to date has been in patients with chronic disorders such as chronic posttraumatic

J. Douglas Bremner is Associate Professor of Psychiatry and Radiology, Emory University School of Medicine, and is affiliated with the Atlanta Veterans Administration Medical Center, Atlanta, GA.

Address correspondence to: J. Douglas Bremner, MD, PET Center/Nuclear Medicine, Emory University Hospital, 1364 Clifton Road, Atlanta, GA 30322 (E-mail: jdbremn@emory.edu).

[Haworth co-indexing entry note]: "Effects of Traumatic Stress on Brain Structure and Function: Relevance to Early Responses to Trauma." Bremner, J. Douglas. Co-published simultaneously in *Journal of Trauma & Dissociation* (The Haworth Medical Press, an imprint of The Haworth Press, Inc.) Vol. 6, No. 2, 2005, pp. 51-68; and: *Acute Reactions to Trauma and Psychotherapy: A Multidisciplinary and International Perspective* (ed: Etzel Cardeña, and Kristin Croyle) The Haworth Medical Press, an imprint of The Haworth Press, Inc., 2005, pp. 51-68. Single or multiple copies of this article are available for a fee from The Haworth Document Delivery Service [1-800-HAWORTH, 9:00 a.m. - 5:00 p.m. (EST). E-mail address: docdelivery@haworthpress.com].

Available online at http://www.haworthpress.com/web/JTD
doi:10.1300/J229v06n02_06

stress disorder (PTSD). Only a few treatment studies have been performed in the early trauma period, and more research in this area is needed. *[Article copies available for a fee from The Haworth Document Delivery Service: 1-800-HAWORTH. E-mail address: <docdelivery@haworthpress.com> Website: <http://www.HaworthPress.com> © 2005 by The Haworth Press, Inc. All rights reserved.]*

**KEYWORDS.** Posttraumatic stress disorder, PTSD, brain, hippocampus

The psychological consequences of acute psychological trauma have long been recognized. In World War I syndromes of "traumatic neurosis" and "shell shock" were initially described. Soldiers were noted to forget their names or where they were on the battlefield; they also developed hyperarousal and extreme fear with reminders of the trauma (Saigh & Bremner, 1999a). Over the course of the 20th century, diagnostic conceptualizations have changed, so that while in earlier versions of the *Diagnostic and Statistical Manual (DSM)*–the American Psychiatric Association's guide for diagnostic criteria, Gross Stress Reaction was conceived of as a temporary response, by the time Posttraumatic Stress Disorder (PTSD) was included in the *DSM* in 1980, the effects of stress were felt to be long-lasting in a subgroup of patients. Since the time when PTSD was first officially recognized, there has been increased awareness of the potentially debilitating effects of traumatic stress that recently culminated in the widespread recognition and awareness of the possible long-term effects of the attack on the World Trade Center on the U.S. society at large. In spite of the chilling images and heart-rending stories of the victims and the survivors of the WTC attack, little is currently known about the acute and chronic effects of these types of traumatic stressors. Studies performed in other populations such as abuse survivors and combat veterans may provide some insight into the potential long-term consequences of traumatic stress, and help to guide future research on the acute effects of trauma.

Posttraumatic stress disorder (PTSD) is characterized by specific symptoms that develop following exposure to a "threat to the life of oneself or others accompanied by intense fear, horror, or helplessness" (American Psychiatric Association, 2000). Symptoms of PTSD include intrusions (intrusive memories, flashbacks, feeling worse with reminders of the trauma, nightmares), avoidance (avoidance of thinking about the event, avoidance of reminders, decreased concentration, amnesia, feeling cut off from others, sense of foreshortened future) and hyper-arousal (increased startle, hyperarousal, hypervigilance, decreased sleep). Although earlier versions of the *DSM* had acute and chronic PTSD, the most recent version of the *DSM* included only a requirement of two months duration of symptoms to diagnose PTSD. Of note is that a sub-stantial proportion of persons with PTSD continue to have chronic symptoms. For example, 30% of Vietnam combat veterans will meet criteria for PTSD early after exposure to trauma; however about half (15%) of those patients go on to develop chronic PTSD (Kulka et al., 1990). There is some evidence that early interventions can prevent the development of chronic PTSD. On a biological level, early modifica-tions while memories are being consolidated are felt to be most useful, before the memories become strongly engraved and more resistant to further intervention.

Other psychiatric disorders are associated with trauma exposure, in-cluding depression, anxiety, dissociative disorders, eating disorders, and alcohol and substance abuse. Acute Stress Disorder captures the early aftermath (first month) after trauma exposure and includes symp-toms of both PTSD and dissociation. There is considerable overlap or "comorbidity" in trauma patients with these diagnoses. Bremner (2002) has argued that these disorders should be considered as part of a *trauma spectrum* of psychiatric disorders, all sharing in common a stress-in-duced alteration in brain circuits and systems. This paper reviews alter-ations in brain structure and function following trauma in the context of understanding early responses to trauma. More comprehensive reviews of PTSD in general (Saigh & Bremner, 1999b) and the neurobiology of stress and PTSD have been presented elsewhere (Bremner, 2002; Bremner, Southwick, & Charney, 1999b).

## EFFECTS OF TRAUMATIC STRESS ON PHYSICAL HEALTH

Stress appears to have lasting effects on physical health that may be compounded by the symptoms of PTSD (Friedman, Charney, & Deutch, 1995). The stress hormones cortisol and adrenaline mediate many of the negative long-term consequences of stress on the body. Although cortisol released during the time of the life-threatening danger is one of the most important factors that helps survival, it may have long-term negative ef-fects on several organ systems (Sapolsky, 1996). Many of these effects are mediated by increased release of the body's hormonal systems–including cortisol–that act like fire alarms to mobilize the resources of the body in life-threatening situations. The hormones cortisol and adrenaline travel throughout the body and brain and have a number of actions that are critical for survival during life-threatening danger.

The parts of the body that are most sensitive to the "wear and tear" effects of stress over time are (logically enough) those areas that are mobilized during the stress response (McEwen & Stellar, 1993; Seeman, Singer, Rowe, Horwitz, & McEwen, 1997). Adrenaline has a number of actions in the body, including stimulation of the heart to beat more rapidly and squeeze harder with each contraction, whereas norepinephrine acting in the brain helps to sharpen focus and stimulate memory. Blood pressure increases to increase blood flow and delivery of oxygen and glucose (necessary energy stores for the cells of the body to cope with the increased demand). There is a shunting of blood flow away from the gut and toward the brain and the muscles. The spleen increases the release of red blood cells that allows the body to send more oxygen to the muscles. The liver converts glycogen to glucose, the type of sugar that can be immediately used. Breathing becomes heavy, so that extra oxygen can get to the lungs, and the pupils dilate for better vision. Release of endogenous opiates acts on the brain to dull our sense of pain, so that the pain of a physical injury incurred during an attack does not impair our ability to escape from the situation. More delayed stress responses include release of cortisol that dampens the immune system, and conversion of fat to glucose in the liver.

These stress hormones can have more insidious, detrimental long-term effects. For instance, excessive levels of cortisol result in a thinning of the lining of the stomach that increases the risk for gastric ulcers. Cortisol also results in a thinning of the bones that increases the risk of osteoporosis and bone fractures in older people, or impairment in reproduction. Other diseases that have been linked to stress include heart disease, diabetes, and asthma. Stress also impairs the immune system, which can lead to an increase in infections and possibly even increased rates of cancer. Chronic stress with decreased blood flow to the intestines can result in chronic ulcers.

There is also some preliminary evidence that stress and possibly PTSD and/or other stress-related disorders like depression are associated with an increased risk of heart disease. Cortisol released during stress acts to increase blood pressure, heart rate, and cholesterol, and raises blood levels of adrenaline (norepinephrine and epinephrine) (McEwen & Stellar, 1993). Increased sympathoadrenal function has been shown to affect cardiovascular function in several ways, including increasing heart rate and blood pressure, increasing endothelial injury, platelet aggregation, and vascular reactivity. Studies in animals in fact have found direct evidence for the damaging effects of stress on blood vessels in the heart and accelerated cardiovascular disease (Rozanski, Blumenthal, & Kaplan, 1999). Some studies have directly linked changes in platelet aggregation and vascular reactivity with depression (Musselman, Evans, & Nemeroff, 1998).

The effects of stress on physical health appear to be caused by a disruption of the balance or homeostasis between different organs of the body. According to this model, stress results in long-term wear and tear that leads to poor health and an increased risk for mortality. Some authors (McEwen & Stellar, 1993) have argued for such a multi-system approach to understanding the effects of stress on the individual, which incorporates neurological/cognitive, hormonal, cardiovascular, and metabolic parameters. This theoretical background has been used to construct a series of assessments of a variety of physical parameters related to endocrine, metabolic, neurological, cognitive, and cardiovascular parameters (Seeman et al., 1997). Using this data the authors constructed an index of "allostatic load," which they hypothesized is related to the long-term effects of stress on physiology. They found that this index was associated with poorer long-term cognitive and physical function, as well as increased risk for cardiovascular disease, in a longitudinal study of an aging population (Seeman et al., 1997).

## NEURAL CIRCUITS AND STRUCTURES IN THE STRESS RESPONSE

Neuroimaging has provided powerful information about neural circuits involved in the stress response (Bremner, 2002). The first neuroimaging study in PTSD was performed using magnetic resonance imaging (MRI) to measure the volume of the hippocampus, a brain area that plays an important role in new learning and memory (Bremner et al., 1995). This research was based on animal studies showing that stress was associated with damage to the CA3 region of the hippocampus. Mechanisms proposed for the effects of stress on the hippocampus include elevated levels of the stress hormone cortisol or excitatory amino acids causing damage to the hippocampus (Sapolsky, 1996), stress induced reductions in brain-derived neurotrophic factor (Nibuya, Morinobu, & Duman, 1995) and stress-induced inhibition of neurogenesis (Gould, Tanapat, McEwen, Flugge, & Fuchs, 1998). Administration of the anti-epileptic medication phenytoin (Dilantin), blocked the negative effects of stress on the hippocampus, probably acting through modulation of the excitatory amino acid system (Watanabe, Gould, Cameron, Daniels, & McEwen, 1992). Administration of selective serotonin reuptake inhibitors (SSRIs) also prevented the stress-induced inhibition of neurogenesis and promoted neurogenesis in the hippocampus (Duman, Heninger, & Nestler, 1997). A study of combat veterans with PTSD showed deficits in paragraph recall (Wechsler Memory Scale Delayed Recall) and new word learning (Selective Reminding Test) that were correlated with decreased hippocampal volume (Bremner et al., 1993). Findings of deficits in hippocampal-based verbal declarative memory have been replicated in several studies of PTSD related to combat and abuse (Bremner, 2002). In a study of Vietnam combat veterans, there was an 8% decrease in MRI-based measurement of right hippocampal volume in patients with PTSD ($N = 26$) in comparison to matched controls ($N = 22$; $p < 0.05$). Decreases in right hippocampal volume in the PTSD patients were associated with deficits in short-term memory as measured by the WMS-Logical Memory, percent retention subcomponent ($r = 0.64$; $p < 0.05$) (Bremner et al., 1995). Findings of smaller hippocampal volume have now been replicated several times in the published literature, with findings of a 26% reduction in bilateral hippocampal volume in combat-related PTSD (Gurvits et al., 1996), a 12% reduction in left hippocampal volume in abuse-related PTSD (Bremner, Randall et al., 1997), and a 5% reduction in left hippocampal volume in women sexually abused as children, most of whom had PTSD (Stein, Koverola, Hanna, Torchia, & McClarty, 1997). Other studies in combat veterans have found reductions (Gilbertson et al., 2002; Villarreal et al., 2002) although not all studies consistently showed reductions (Schuff et al., 2001).

Several questions that arose from these early studies were how long it takes for hippocampal damage to develop, and whether the effects are reversible. Findings from animal studies suggest that the effects revert to normal; this suggests that for changes in hippocampal structure to be seen in human subjects there is a need for chronic ongoing stressors. In fact, recent studies showing no hippocampal volume reduction in children with PTSD (Carrion et al., 2001; De Bellis, Hall, Boring, Frustaci, & Moritz, 2001; De Bellis et al., 1999) and new-onset PTSD (Bonne et al., 2001) suggest that hippocampal volume changes are primarily seen in chronic, severe PTSD. However, a process that leads to hippocampal volume changes with chronic PTSD likely begins with the initial acute trauma. Other factors, such as the chronic stress of PTSD symptoms or increased vulnerability to re-traumatization, then contribute to hippo-campal volume changes, perhaps through an inhibition of neurogenesis or other factors. We do have some preliminary information on the potential for reversibility in human studies that is relevant to the acute trauma response. In an unpublished study, we treated 23 PTSD patients for one year with the SSRI paroxetine, and found a 5% increase in hippocampal volume and a 35% improvement in hippocampal-based verbal declarative memory function (measured with the Wechsler Memory Scale). These findings raise the question of whether pre-treatment or early treatment with SSRIs may prevent the development of neurological deficits from acute trauma. Alternatively, other authors have argued that stress does not lead to hippocampal damage. Rather, genetic predisposition to smaller hippocampal volume and lower memory function leads to a vulnerability to PTSD (Gilbertson et al., 2002).

Functional neuroimaging studies have also started to map a neural circuitry for PTSD. Yohimbine induced increases in noradrenergic release and PTSD symptoms resulted in decreased metabolism in hippocampus as well as other areas including medial prefrontal and orbitofrontal cortex (Bremner, Innis et al., 1997). Several studies have used PET measurement of brain blood flow with radioactive water ($H_2[^{15}O]$) in conjunction with provocation of PTSD symptoms and traumatic recall using traumatic reminders such as combat slides and sounds and traumatic personalized scripts. One uncontrolled study that looked at PTSD patients with a range of traumas ($N = 8$) exposed to trauma-related scripts found an increase in brain blood flow in limbic regions (right amygdala, insula, orbitofrontal cortex, and anterior cingulate), and decreased blood flow in middle temporal and left inferior frontal cortex (Rauch et al., 1996).

In another study, 10 Vietnam veterans with PTSD and 10 Vietnam veterans without PTSD were exposed to combat-related slides and sounds in conjunction with PET imaging. Vietnam veterans with combat-related PTSD (but not non-PTSD veterans) demonstrated a decrease in blood flow in the medial prefrontal cortex (Brodmann's area 25, or subcallosal gyrus) and middle temporal cortex (auditory cortex) during exposure to combat-related slides and sounds, with relative increases in activity in lingual gyrus (posterior parahippocampus), and posterior cingulate, as well as left inferior parietal and left motor cortex, and dorsal pons (Bremner, Staib et al., 1999).

Exposure to neutral and combat trauma related pictures (without sounds) and mental imagery in combat veterans with ($N = 7$) and without ($N = 7$) PTSD showed increased blood flow in anterior cingulate during combat versus neutral imagery in PTSD. Blood flow was also increased in right amygdala during combat imagery versus exposure to combat-related pictures in PTSD, while controls (but not patients) had increased blood flow in orbitofrontal and medial prefrontal cortex during these conditions. PTSD patients (but not controls) also had decreased blood flow in middle temporal and left inferior frontal cortex during exposure to traumatic mental imagery (Shin et al., 1997). Other studies have shown decreased medial prefrontal function in combat-related PTSD during exposure to combat-related sounds (Liberzon et al., 1999).

Several studies have now examined neural correlates of childhood abuse-related PTSD. We measured brain blood flow with PET and $H_2[^{15}O]$ during exposure to personalized scripts of childhood sexual abuse. Twenty-two women with a history of childhood sexual abuse underwent injection of $H_2[^{15}O]$ followed by positron emission tomography (PET) imaging of the brain while listening to neutral and traumatic (personalized childhood sexual abuse events) scripts. Brain blood flow during exposure to traumatic versus neutral scripts was compared between sexually abused women with ($N = 10$) and without PTSD ($N = 12$). Memories of childhood sexual abuse were associated with greater increases in blood flow in portions of anterior prefrontal cortex (superior and middle frontal gyri-areas 6 and 9), posterior cingulate (area 31), and motor cortex in sexually abused women with PTSD compared to sexually abused women without PTSD. Abuse memories were associated with alterations in blood flow in medial prefrontal cortex, with decreased blood flow in subcallosal gyrus–area 25, and a failure of activation in anterior cingulated–area 32. There was also decreased blood flow in right hippocampus, fusiform/inferior temporal gyrus, supramarginal gyrus, and visual association cortex in PTSD relative to non-PTSD women (Bremner, Narayan et al., 1999). This study replicated findings of decreased function in medial prefrontal cortex and increased function in posterior cingulate in combat-related PTSD during exposure to combat-related slides and sounds.

Another study looked at eight women with childhood sexual abuse and PTSD and eight women with abuse without PTSD using PET during exposure to script-driven imagery of childhood abuse. The authors found increases in orbitofrontal cortex and anterior temporal pole in both groups of subjects, with greater increases in these areas in the PTSD group. PTSD patients showed a relative failure of anterior cingulate activation compared to controls. The PTSD patients (but not controls) showed decreased blood flow in anteromedial portions of prefrontal cortex and left inferior frontal gyrus (Shin et al., 1999).

Preliminary studies from our group found decreased hippocampal and medial prefrontal cortical function during remembrance of emotionally valenced words (e.g., "blood," "stench") in women with abuse-related PTSD (Bremner, Vythilingam, Vermetten, Southwick, McGlashan, Staib et al., 2003). In a second study, we utilized encoding of a paragraph as a probe of hippocampal function. This was based on the fact that we have consistently demonstrated deficits in paragraph recall in PTSD, the PET literature showing more consistent activation with encoding versus retrieval tasks, which we have reviewed elsewhere (Bremner et al., 2001), as well as our own pilot testing that showed greater activation with encoding than retrieval. PET imaging in conjunction with the performance of hippocampal-based verbal declarative memory tasks was performed in women with a history of early childhood sexual abuse with ($N = 10$) and without ($N = 12$) PTSD. Hippocampal volume was measured with magnetic resonance imaging (MRI) in three subject groups: women with early childhood sexual abuse and PTSD, women with early abuse without PTSD, and women without early abuse or PTSD. A failure of left hippocampal activation ($F = 14.94$; $df = 1,20$; $p < .001$) and 16% smaller volume of the hippocampus was seen in women with abuse and PTSD compared to women with abuse without PTSD. Abused PTSD women also had a 19% smaller hippocampal volume relative to women without abuse or PTSD (Bremner, Vythilingam, Vermetten, Southwick, McGlashan, Nazeer et al., 2003).

These studies did not find consistent activation of the amygdala, which is known to play a critical role in fear responses (Davis, 1992). Rauch et al. (2000) did find increased amygdala activation in PTSD with exposure to masked fearful faces. In subsequent studies from our group we have further mapped the neural correlates of PTSD using PET imaging in conjunction with the conditioned fear paradigm. In the conditioned fear paradigm, repeated pairing of an aversive unconditioned stimulus (e.g., electric shock; US) with a neutral conditioned stimulus (e.g., bright light; CS), results in a conditioned fear response to the light alone. Animal studies have shown that the amygdala plays a critical role in acquisition of conditioned fear responses, while the medial prefrontal cortex (including anterior cingulate), through inhibition of amygdala responsiveness, has been hypothesized to play a role in extinction of fear responses. In a study of PTSD we found that patients had increased left amygdala activation with fear acquisition, and decreased medial prefrontal (anterior cingulate) function during extinction, relative to controls. These findings implicate amygdala and medial prefrontal cortex (anterior cingulate) in the acquisition and extinction of fear responses, respectively, in PTSD. Another PET study with the Stroop paradigm showed a failure of anterior cingulate activation in PTSD.

Other studies have found deficits in anterior cingulate and medial prefrontal cortex in childhood trauma populations. One study used single voxel proton magnetic resonance spectroscopy (proton MRS) to measure relative concentration of N-acetylaspartate and creatinine (a marker of neuronal viability) in the anterior cingulate of 11 children with maltreatment-related PTSD and 11 controls. The authors found a reduction in the ratio of N-acetylaspartate to creatinine in PTSD relative to controls (De Bellis, Keshavan, Spencer, & Hall, 2000).

A number of PET studies have now implicated medial prefrontal cortex in both normal and pathological responses to stress and emotion. In the PET studies conducted by our group there was a failure of activation of anterior cingulate and decreased blood flow in medial prefrontal cortex (subcallosal gyrus) during exposure to traumatic stimuli in PTSD. PET studies in normal subjects using a variety of paradigms to stimulate intense emotions have consistently demonstrated activation of the anterior cingulate (areas 32 and 24). Human subjects with lesions of medial prefrontal cortical areas (e.g., the famous case of Phineas Gage) have deficits in interpretation of emotional situations that are accompanied by impairments in social relatedness. Lesions of this area in animals result in impairments in mounting the peripheral glucocorticoid and sympathetic response to stress (Bremner, 2002).

Findings from imaging studies may also be relevant to the failure of extinction to fear responding that is characteristic of PTSD and other anxiety disorders. Recent evidence suggests that extinction is mediated by cortical inhibition of amygdala responsiveness. Medial prefrontal cortex (area 25) or adjacent medial prefrontal regions (anterior cingulate, areas 24 and 32, and orbitofrontal cortex) have inhibitory connections to the amygdala that play a role in extinction of fear responding, an important component of the symptom profile of PTSD. PET studies in PTSD during traumatic reminders reviewed earlier showed decreased blood flow of the medial prefrontal cortex (area 25), with failure of activation of anterior cingulate and medial orbitofrontal cortex. Based on these findings, we previously argued that anterior cingulate (area 32) activation represents a "normal" brain response to traumatic stimuli that serves to inhibit feelings of fearfulness when there is no true threat. Failure of activation in this area and/or decreased blood flow in adjacent medial prefrontal cortex (area 25) in PTSD may lead to increased fearfulness that is not appropriate for the context, a behavioral response that is highly characteristic of patients with PTSD.

Plasticity in the hippocampus may also be relevant to the development of psychopathology following exposure to acute traumas. Preclinical studies show that there is a window during which modification of traumatic memories may affect long-term outcome. In animals who have encoded a traumatic memory, lesions of the hippocampus within the first month will cancel the traumatic memory. However, after a month, hippocampal lesions have no effect on the traumatic memory. These studies suggest that there is a critical window of memory consolidation during which memories are stored within the hippocampus and are susceptible to memory consolidation; after this time period memories are stored in the cerebral cortex and are strongly engraved and more resistant to modification (Bremner, Southwick et al., 1999b). These findings suggest that early interventions are important to prevent the development of strongly engraved memories that will maintain chronic PTSD. However, as discussed later, we do not have enough evidence to support specific treatments for PTSD.

## *ACUTE AND CHRONIC NEUROBIOLOGICAL RESPONSES TO TRAUMA*

Much of our knowledge related to the acute trauma response is based on anecdotal or clinically-based information. Military psychiatrists have long treated acutely traumatized soldiers with benzodiazepines or chlorpromazine on the battlefield and kept them close to the front lines. They knew from experience that if you removed a soldier from the front lines, it would be almost impossible to get them to go back. These military psychiatrists were in effect practicing a form of desensitization therapy. In other words, exposure to the front lines promoted extinction of fear responses to the traumatic stimulus, in this case reminders of combat.

Little is known about the acute neurobiological trauma response. Because the acute phase of the trauma response is generally felt to be limited to three months or less, it is difficult to obtain the necessary funding and investigational review board approval, and to plan and coordinate data collection, in the aftermath of large-scale disasters such as the WTC attack. For these reasons most studies have been conducted in individuals with chronic PTSD who are a year or more past their original trauma. Although these studies have their limitations in reference to understanding and treating the acute trauma response, they do represent an important starting point for this area of investigation.

Comparing the effects of treatment during the acute and chronic phases of the trauma response may provide insight into early responses to trauma (Mellman, Byers, & Augenstein, 1998). Robert et al. (1999) compared imipramine to chloral hydrate for children who were acute burn victims. The authors found that imipramine treatment led to a significant improvement in psychiatric symptoms compared to chloral hydrate (Robert, Blakeney, Villarreal, Rosenberg, & Meyer, 1999). Gelpin et al. found that treatment of acute trauma survivors presenting to an emergency room with the benzodiazepine medication, alprazolam, when compared to placebo, actually made patients worse in terms of long-term development of PTSD (Gelpin, Bonne, Peri, Brandes, & Shalev, 1996). Pitman et al. (2002) showed that the noradrenergic beta receptor blocker, propanolol, administered in the emergency room to acute trauma victims, blocked the development of psychophysiological responses, although there was only a modest effect on PTSD symptoms.

Studies by Foa and others (Foa et al., 1999; Meadows & Foa, 1999) found cognitive behavioral therapies for rape victims to be more efficacious if they are delivered during the acute phase of the trauma response. Also reviewed in this volume are studies showing that other types of behavioral treatments such as psychological debriefing or critical incident stress debriefing which are offered to acute trauma victims, have been found in several studies to actually worsen outcome relative to no treatment at all. Although there is a natural tendency to want to do something for the acute trauma victim, these studies should give us pause before we apply untested treatments to acute trauma victims.

These studies also suggest that there is a window of brain plasticity during the phase of the acute trauma response when there is a greater potential to affect the final outcome (for better or for worse) in terms of chronic PTSD. Preclinical studies provide a model for the mechanism of how this phenomenon may occur. For example, as noted earlier, lesions of the hippocampus in the first 30 days after an aversive learning event (i.e., the learning of a negative memory) will erase the memory. However after that time window, the memories are strongly engraved and more resistant to modification. This may be related to the transfer of memories to long-term storage in the cerebral cortex. Stress sensitization of neurochemical systems may also explain the change from acute to chronic trauma responses. After initial stress there is release of stress hormones and neurotransmitters including cortisol and norepinephrine.

With chronic and repeated stress there is a potentiated release of, for example, norepinephrine following exposure to subsequent stressors. This process, called stress sensitization, may explain the transition from the acute to the chronic stress response.

Another phenomenon that is relevant to understanding early responses to stress is extinction. We still do not understand the processes that are involved in turning off the fear response, which is a critical factor determining who will and will not develop chronic PTSD responses. However preliminary animal and human imaging data suggests that dysfunction in the medial prefrontal cortex with a failure to inhibit amygdala function may mediate in part this process. Repeated stress may also cause changes in brain areas such as the hippocampus, in a manner analogous to kindling, which is used as a model for understanding the development of epilepsy. Changes in the hippocampus may actually help to promote and maintain symptoms of the disorder.

Understanding the acute trauma response may be useful in the development of new treatments that can reverse early PTSD or even block the development of PTSD. Preclinical studies showing that stress-induced stimulation of noradrenergic function may modulate the laying down of traumatic memories have stimulated interest in the use of agents that may block noradrenergic function for the treatment of acute trauma. For example, animal studies have shown that pharmacological blockade of the beta receptor in the amygdala prevents the laying down of emotionally aversive memory. As mentioned earlier, Pitman and colleagues (2002) treated patients in the emergency room with the noradrenergic beta blocker, propanolol, with hours of experiencing trauma, and continued treatment for several weeks later. The investigators found that propanolol did not lead to a significant reduction in PTSD symptoms compared to placebo; however there was a decrease in conditioned physiologic responses to traumatic reminders (Pitman et al., 2002). This study seemed to suggest that propanolol interfered with the acquisition of conditioned responses, but not the development of core PTSD symptoms per se. Theories of PTSD as related to kindling underlie in part the application of medications used for epilepsy, like tegretol and valproic acid. These agents have effects on mood and have been shown to be efficacious in open-label trials in PTSD. One 12 week placebo-controlled trial of lamotrigine showed improvement on both re-experiencing and avoidance/numbing symptoms (Hertzberg et al., 1999). Dilantin is particularly of interest, since it is efficacious in epilepsy and, as reviewed earlier in this paper, has been shown in animal studies to block the negative effects of stress on hippocampal morphology. Animal studies have also shown that treatment with corticotropin releasing factor (CRF) an Nemeroff, 1999; Habib et al., 2000). This has prompted an interest in developing clinical trials for acute trauma victims.

There is also evidence from animal studies that stress is associated with alterations in the serotonin system. Pretreatment with serotonin reuptake inhibitors and tricyclics before stress exposure prevented the development of chronic behavioral disturbances. Also SSRIs prevent stress-induced inhibition of neurogenesis, or the growth of neurons, in the hippocampus. Hippocampal dysfunction may contribute to both cognitive dysfunction and emotional dysregulation in PTSD. There also may be a window of opportunity in the acute aftermath of stress when these effects can be blocked or reversed. This leads us to the speculation that SSRIs given to acute trauma victims, or pre-administered to individuals at risk of stress, may prevent PTSD.

## CONCLUSIONS

This paper has reviewed alterations in brain structure and function in PTSD in the context of early stress responses. Stress is associated with an acute physiological response, which includes release of stress hormones and neurotransmitters including cortisol and norepinephrine. The physiological stress response also has negative long-term effects on physical health, which is at least partially mediated by these hormones and neurotransmitters, conferring an increased risk for heart disease and other disorders. Acute stress responses following exposure to chronic stressors are associated with a potentiated release of norepinephrine. Difficulties in conducting biological research in acute trauma victims have resulted in a situation where most of our knowledge is based on studies in patients with chronic PTSD. These studies have implicated brain regions including the medial prefrontal cortex, hippocampus, and amygdala in the neural circuitry of PTSD. There may be a window of opportunity in the acute aftermath of stress where the detrimental effects of stress on these brain circuits and systems can be reversed or blocked, leading to the prevention of PTSD. Future studies are needed to assess the early response to trauma and longitudinal course of the development of PTSD, both in terms of neurobiology and treatment.

# REFERENCES

American Psychiatric Association. (2000). *Diagnostic and statistical manual of mental disorders, 4th ed.*, text revision. Washington, DC: Author.

Arborelius, L., Owens, M.J., Plotsky, P.M., & Nemeroff, C.B. (1999). The role of corticotropin-releasing factor in depression and anxiety disorders. *Journal of Endocrinology, 160,* 1-12.

Bonne, O., Brandes, D., Gilboa, A., Gomori, J.M., Shenton, M.E., Pitman, R.K., & Shalev, A.Y. (2001). Longitudinal MRI study of hippocampal volume in trauma survivors with PTSD. *American Journal of Psychiatry, 158,* 1248-1251.

Bremner, J.D. (2002). *Does stress damage the brain? Understanding trauma-related disorders from a mind-body perspective.* New York: W.W. Norton.

Bremner, J.D., Innis, R.B., Ng, C.K., Staib, L., Duncan, J., Bronen, R., Zubal, G., Rich, D., Krystal, J.H., Dey, H., Soufer, R., & Charney, D.S. (1997). PET measurement of cerebral metabolic correlates of yohimbine administration in posttraumatic stress disorder. *Archives of General Psychiatry, 54,* 246-256.

Bremner, J.D., Narayan, M., Staib, L.H., Southwick, S.M., McGlashan, T., & Charney, D.S. (1999). Neural correlates of memories of childhood sexual abuse in women with and without posttraumatic stress disorder. *American Journal of Psychiatry, 156,* 1787-1795.

Bremner, J.D., Randall, P.R., Scott, T.M., Bronen, R.A., Delaney, R.C., Seibyl, J.P., Southwick, S.M., McCarthy, G., Charney, D.S., & Innis, R.B. (1995). MRI-based measurement of hippocampal volume in posttraumatic stress disorder. *American Journal of Psychiatry, 152,* 973-981.

Bremner, J.D., Randall, P.R., Vermetten, E., Staib, L., Bronen, R.A., Mazure, C.M., Capelli, S., McCarthy, G., Innis, R.B., & Charney, D.S. (1997). MRI-based measurement of hippocampal volume in posttraumatic stress disorder related to childhood physical and sexual abuse: A preliminary report. *Biological Psychiatry, 41,* 23-32.

Bremner, J.D., Scott, T.M., Delaney, R.C., Southwick, S.M., Mason, J.W., Johnson, D.R., Innis, R.B., McCarthy, G., & Charney, D.S. (1993). Deficits in short-term memory in post-traumatic stress disorder. *American Journal of Psychiatry, 150,* 1015-1019.

Bremner, J.D., Soufer, R., McCarthy, G., Delaney, R.C., Staib, L.H., Duncan, J.S., & Charney, D.S. (2001). Gender differences in cognitive and neural correlates of remembrance of emotional words. *Psychopharmacology Bulletin, 35,* 55-87.

Bremner, J.D., Southwick, S.M., & Charney, D.S. (1999). The neurobiology of posttraumatic stress disorder: An integration of animal and human research. In P.A. Saigh & J. D. Bremner (Eds.), *Posttraumatic stress disorder: A comprehensive text* (pp. 103-143). Needham Heights, MA: Allyn & Bacon.

Bremner, J.D., Staib, L., Kaloupek, D., Southwick, S.M., Soufer, R., & Charney, D.S. (1999). Positron emission tomographic (PET)-based measurement of cerebral blood flow correlates of traumatic reminders in Vietnam combat veterans with and without posttraumatic stress disorder (PTSD). *Biological Psychiatry, 45,* 806-816.

Bremner, J.D., Vythilingam, M., Vermetten, E., Southwick, S.M., McGlashan, T., Nazeer, A., Khan, S., Vaccarino, L.V., Soufer, R., Garg, P., Ng, C.K., Staib, L.H.,

Duncan, J.S., & Charney, D.S. (2003). MRI and PET study of deficits in hippo-campal structure and function in women with childhood sexual abuse and post-traumatic stress disorder (PTSD). *American Journal of Psychiatry, 160,* 924-932.

Bremner, J.D., Vythilingam, M., Vermetten, E., Southwick, S.M., McGlashan, T., Staib, L., Soufer, R., & Charney, D.S. (2003). Neural correlates of declarative memory for emotionally valenced words in women with posttraumatic stress disorder (PTSD) related to early childhood sexual abuse. *Biological Psychiatry, 53,* 289-299.

Carrion, V.G., Weems, C.F., Eliez, S., Patwardhan, A., Brown, W., Ray, R.D., & Reiss, A.L. (2001). Attenuation of frontal asymmetry in pediatric posttraumatic stress disorder. *Biological Psychiatry, 50,* 943-951.

Davis, M. (1992). The role of the amygdala in fear and anxiety. *Annual Review of Neuroscience, 15,* 353-375.

De Bellis, M.D., Hall, J., Boring, A.M., Frustaci, K., & Moritz, G. (2001). A pilot longitudinal study of hippocampal volumes in pediatric maltreatment-related posttraumatic stress disorder. *Biological Psychiatry, 50,* 305-309.

De Bellis, M.D., Keshavan, M.S., Clark, D.B., Casey, B.J., Giedd, J.N., Boring, A.M., Frustaci, K., & Ryan, N.D. (1999). A.E. Bennett Research Award: Developmental traumatology: Part II. Brain development. *Biological Psychiatry, 45,* 1271-1284.

De Bellis, M.D., Keshavan, M.S., Spencer, S., & Hall, J. (2000). N-acetylaspartate concentration in the anterior cingulate of maltreated children and adolescents with PTSD. *American Journal of Psychiatry, 157,* 1175-1177.

Duman, R.S., Heninger, G.R., & Nestler, E.J. (1997). A molecular and cellular theory of depression. *Archives of General Psychiatry, 54,* 597-606.

Foa, E.B., Davidson, J.R.T., Frances, A., Culpepper, L., Ross, R., & Ross, D. (1999). The expert consensus guideline series: Treatment of posttraumatic stress disorder. *Journal of Clinical Psychiatry, 60,* 4-76.

Friedman, M.J., Charney, D.S., & Deutch, A.Y. (1995). *Neurobiological and clinical consequences of stress: From normal adaptation to PTSD.* New York: Raven Press.

Gelpin, E., Bonne, O., Peri, T., Brandes, D., & Shalev, A.Y. (1996). Treatment of recent trauma survivors with benzodiazepines: A prospective study. *Journal of Clinical Psychiatry, 57,* 390-394.

Gilbertson, M.W., Shenton, M.E., Ciszewski, A., Kasai, K., Lasko, N.B., Orr, S.P., & Pitman, R.K. (2002). Smaller hippocampal volume predicts pathologic vulnerability to psychological trauma. *Nature Neuroscience, 5,* 1242-1247.

Gould, E., Tanapat, P., McEwen, B.S., Flugge, G., & Fuchs, E. (1998). Proliferation of granule cell precursors in the dentate gyrus of adult monkeys is diminished by stress. *Proceedings of the National Academy of Sciences USA, 95,* 3168-3171.

Gurvits, T.G., Shenton, M.R., Hokama, H., Ohta, H., Lasko, N.B., Gilbertson, M.B., Orr, S.P., Kikinis, R., & Lolesz, F.A. (1996). Magnetic resonance imaging study of hippocampal volume in chronic combat-related posttraumatic stress disorder. *Biological Psychiatry, 40,* 192-199.

Habib, K.E., Weld, K.P., Rice, K.C., Pushkas, J., Champoux, M., Listwak, S., Webster, E.L., Atkinson, A.J., Schulkin, J., Contoreggi, C., Chrousos, G.P., McCann, S.M., Suomi, S.J., Higley, J.D., & Gold, P.W. (2000). Oral administration of a corticotropin-releasing hormone receptor antagonist significantly attenuates behavioral neuroendocrine and autonomic responses to stress in primates. *Proceedings of the National Academy of Sciences USA, 97*, 6079-6084.

Hertzberg, M.A., Butterfield, M.I., Feldman, M.E., Beckham, J.C., Sutherland, S.M., Connor, K.M., & Davidson, J.R. (1999). A preliminary study of lamotrigine for the treatment of posttraumatic stress disorder. *Biological Psychiatry, 45*, 1226-1229.

Kulka, R.A., Schlenger, W.E., Fairbank, J.A., Hough, R.L., Jordan, B.K., Marmar, C.R., & Weiss, D.S. (1990). *Trauma and the Vietnam war generation: Report of findings from the National Vietnam Veterans Readjustment Study.* New York: Brunner/Mazel.

Liberzon, I., Taylor, S.F., Amdur, R., Jung, T.D., Chamberlain, K.R., Minoshima, S., Koeppe, R.A., & Fig, L.M. (1999). Brain activation in PTSD in response to trauma-related stimuli. *Biological Psychiatry, 45*, 817-826.

McEwen, B.S., & Stellar, E. (1993). Stress and the individual: Mechanisms leading to disease. *Archives of Internal Medicine, 153*, 2093-2101.

Meadows, E.A., & Foa, E.B. (1999). Cognitive-behavioral treatment of traumatized adults. In P.A. Saigh, & J. D. Bremner (Eds.), *Posttraumatic Stress Disorder: A comprehensive text* (pp. 376-390). Needham Heights, MA: Allyn & Bacon.

Mellman, T.A., Byers, P.M., & Augenstein, J.S. (1998). Pilot evaluation of hypnotic medication during acute traumatic stress response. *Journal of Traumatic Stress, 11*, 563-569.

Musselman, D.L., Evans, D.L., & Nemeroff, C.B. (1998). The relationship of depression to cardiovascular disease. *Archives of General Psychiatry, 55*, 580-592.

Nibuya, M., Morinobu, S., & Duman, R.S. (1995). Regulation of BDNF and trkB mRNA in rat brain by chronic electroconvulsive seizure and antidepressant drug treatments. *Journal of Neuroscience, 15*, 7539-7547.

Pitman, R.K., Sanders, K.M., Zusman, R.M., Healy, A.R., Cheema, F., Lasko, N.B., Cahill, L., & Orr, S.P. (2002). Pilot study of secondary prevention of posttraumatic stress disorder with propranolol. *Biological Psychiatry, 51*, 189-192.

Rauch, S.L., van der Kolk, B.A., Fisler, R.E., Alpert, N.M., Orr, S.P., Savage, C.R., Fischman, A.J., Jenike, M.A., & Pitman, R.K. (1996). A symptom provocation study of posttraumatic stress disorder using positron emission tomography and script driven imagery. *Archives of General Psychiatry, 53*, 380-387.

Rauch, S.L., Whalen, P.J., Shin, L.M., McInerney, S.C., Macklin, M.L., Lasko, N.B., Orr, S.P., & Pitman, R.K. (2000). Exaggerated amygdala response to masked facial stimuli in posttraumatic stress disorder: A functional MRI study. *Biological Psychiatry, 47*, 769-776.

Robert, R., Blakeney, P.E., Villarreal, C., Rosenberg, L., & Meyer, W.J. (1999). Imipramine treatment in pediatric burn patients with symptoms of acute stress disorder: A pilot study. *Journal of the American Academy of Child & Adolescent Psychiatry, 38*, 873-882.

Rozanski, A., Blumenthal, J.A., & Kaplan, J. (1999). Impact of psychological factors on the pathogenesis of cardiovascular disease and implications for therapy. *Circulation, 99*, 2192-2217.

Saigh, P.A., & Bremner, J.D. (1999a). The history of posttraumatic stress disorder. In P.A. Saigh & J. D. Bremner (Eds.), *Posttraumatic Stress Disorder: A comprehensive text* (pp. 1-17). Needham Heights, MA: Allyn & Bacon.

Saigh, P.A., & Bremner, J.D. (1999b). *Posttraumatic Stress Disorder: A comprehensive text.* Needham Heights, MA: Allyn & Bacon.

Sapolsky, R.M. (1996). Why stress is bad for your brain. *Science, 273,* 749-750.

Schuff, N., Neylan, T.C., Lenoci, M.A., Du, A.T., Weiss, D.S., Marmar, C.R., & Weiner, M.W. (2001). Decreased hippocampal N-acetylaspartate in the absence of atrophy in posttraumatic stress disorder. *Biological Psychiatry, 50,* 952-959.

Seeman, T.E., Singer, B.H., Rowe, J.W., Horwitz, R.I., & McEwen, B.S. (1997). Price of adaptation–Allostatic load and its health consequences. MacArthur studies of successful aging. *Archives of Internal Medicine, 157,* 2259-2268.

Shin, L.H., McNally, R.J., Kosslyn, S.M., Thompson, W.L., Rauch, S.L., Alpert, N.M., Metzger, L.J., Lasko, N.B., Orr, S.P., & Pitman, R.K. (1999). Regional cerebral blood flow during script-driven imagery in childhood sexual abuse-related PTSD: A PET investigation. *American Journal of Psychiatry, 156,* 575-584.

Shin, L.M., Kosslyn, S.M., McNally, R.J., Alpert, N.M., Thompson, W.L., Rauch, S.L., Macklin, M.L., & Pitman, R.K. (1997). Visual imagery and perception in posttraumatic stress disorder: A positron emission tomographic investigation. *Archives of General Psychiatry, 54,* 233-237.

Stein, M.B., Koverola, C., Hanna, C., Torchia, M.G., & McClarty, B. (1997). Hippocampal volume in women victimized by childhood sexual abuse. *Psychological Medicine, 27,* 951-959.

Villarreal, G., Hamilton, D.A., Petropoulos, H., Driscoll, I., Rowland, L.M., Griego, J.A., Kodituwakku, P.W., Hart, B.L., Escalona, R., & Brooks, W.M. (2002). Reduced hippocampal volume and total white matter in posttraumatic stress disorder. *Biological Psychiatry, 52,* 119-125.

Watanabe, Y.E., Gould, H., Cameron, D., Daniels, D., & McEwen, B.S. (1992). Phenytoin prevents stress and corticosterone induced atrophy of CA3 pyramidal neurons. *Hippocampus, 2,* 431-436.

# A Snapshot of Terror:
# Acute Posttraumatic Responses
# to the September 11 Attack

Etzel Cardeña, PhD
J. Michael Dennis, PhD
Mark Winkel, PhD
Linda J. Skitka, PhD

**SUMMARY.** This paper reports on acute posttraumatic reactions and forms of coping to the September 11 attack. We conducted a survey within three weeks of the attack on a nationwide, representative sample

Etzel Cardeña is Thorsen Chair of Psychology, Department of Psychology, University of Lund, Lund, Sweden.

J. Michael Dennis is Vice President and Managing Director for the Government and Academic Research Area, Knowledge Networks, Menlo Park, CA.

Mark Winkel is Associate Professor, Department of Psychology and Anthropology, University of Texas-Pan American, Edinburg, TX.

Linda J. Skitka is Professor, Department of Psychology, University of Illinois at Chicago, Chicago, IL.

Address correspondence to: Etzel Cardeña, PhD, Thorsen Chair of Psychology, Department of Psychology, University of Lund, P.O. Box 213, SE-221 00 Lund, Sweden (E-mail: etzel9@yahoo.com).

An earlier version of this paper was presented at the 104th Annual Meeting of the American Psychological Association, Chicago, IL, August 2002.

The authors gratefully acknowledge the editorial assistance of Kristin Croyle, PhD, and Dana Barth.

[Haworth co-indexing entry note]: "A Snapshot of Terror: Acute Posttraumatic Responses to the September 11 Attack." Cardeña, Etzel et al. Co-published simultaneously in *Journal of Trauma & Dissociation* (The Haworth Medical Press, an imprint of The Haworth Press, Inc.) Vol. 6, No. 2, 2005, pp. 69-84; and: *Acute Reactions to Trauma and Psychotherapy: A Multidisciplinary and International Perspective* (ed: Etzel Cardeña, and Kristin Croyle) The Haworth Medical Press, an imprint of The Haworth Press, Inc., 2005, pp. 69-84. Single or multiple copies of this article are available for a fee from The Haworth Document Delivery Service [1-800-HAWORTH, 9:00 a.m. - 5:00 p.m. (EST). E-mail address: docdelivery@haworthpress.com].

of individuals 13 years or older ($N = 3,134$). Measures included the Stanford Acute Stress Reaction Questionnaire (SASRQ), the brief version of the COPE, and questions about demographics and attitudes toward the attackers. Results show that residents of New York City–women, young adults (but not teens), and people recently immigrated into the country–experienced more distress about the attack. There was a positive linear association between hours of watching TV news related to the attack and distress, and a small positive association between hostility toward the perpetrators, TV watching, and distress. Income, religion, education, and ethnicity did not have an effect on distress. Maladaptive coping strategies and TV watching explained considerably more variance than did demographics. Reactions to acute trauma seem to depend on the lack of appropriate coping strategies. The curvilinear relationship between age and posttraumatic distress suggests caution when interpreting previous findings about age and posttraumatic reactions. The association between media exposure, coping styles, and acute distress among teens extends previous findings and deserves further investigation. *[Article copies available for a fee from The Haworth Document Delivery Service: 1-800-HAWORTH. E-mail address: <docdelivery@haworthpress.com> Website: <http://www.HaworthPress.com> © 2005 by The Haworth Press, Inc. All rights reserved.]*

**KEYWORDS.** September 11, acute reactions, media

The present is *always* an awful place to be.

–*The Homebody*, in Tony Kushner's play *Homebody/Kabul (2002)*

## INTRODUCTION

Researchers have paid great attention to the impact of the September 11, 2001, attacks on the psychological health of USA inhabitants. The challenges when conducting research after an unforeseen catastrophe are daunting, and in these circumstances authors typically have to be circumspect about making causal inferences (North & Pfefferbaum, 2002); even so, this research is important and necessary.

At least four major studies on the psychological impact of September 11 were published within a year of the incident. The first ($N = 560$) was a random-digit dialing nationwide survey of adults within a week of the incident (Schuster et al., 2001). Forty-four percent of respondents endorsed at least one symptom of distress for themselves and their children. For adults, being a female, nonwhite, with prior emotional or mental health problems, living close to the World Trade Center and, generally, in the Northeast, and watching television were associated with distress scores; population density had no effect. Parents with greater levels of distress were more likely to state that their children, especially female, were distressed (35% of children were reported to have at least one symptom). The most commonly reported forms of coping were talking to others, turning to religion, and participating in group activities (Schuster et al., 2001).

Another study used random dialing to survey New York City adult residents ($N = 1008$) between October 16 and November 15 (Galea et al., 2002). The researchers found a rate of about 7.5% probable PTSD and 9.7% probable depression. The following variables were associated with PTSD: female gender, race/ethnicity, living close to the attacks, low social support, previous stressors, directly witnessing the events, panic attack symptoms soon or during the event, having lost possessions, having been involved in rescue efforts, and losing a job because of the attack (Galea et al., 2002). Neither income, education, nor having a friend killed were related to symptoms. In multivariate analyses, only Hispanic ethnicity, multiple stressors, panic attacks, close residency to the attacks, and loss of possessions were significant predictors of probable PTSD (Galea et al., 2002).

A third study conducted a nationwide, representative, web-based survey of adults ($N = 2,273$) 1-2 months after September 11 to evaluate PTSD symptoms and nonspecific psychological distress (Schlenger et al., 2002). In the analysis for the nation as a whole, levels of distress did not vary from what would be expected for a general community sample, except for the New York City (NYC) metropolitan area, which showed greater distress than the rest of the country (prevalence of probable PTSD was 11.2% for NYC vs. 3.6% for other metropolitan areas). Multivariate analyses showed that being female, between 18-29 years of age (no one under 18 years of age was tested), having direct exposure to the attacks, and amount of TV watched predicted PTSD symptoms. Being female, amount of TV watched, and traumatic imagery were related to general distress (Schlenger et al., 2002).

The fourth major research study also used web-based methodology and included part of the same sample as ours (Silver, Holman, McIntosh, Pouli, & Gil-Rivas, 2002). It used a national probability sample of adults ($N =$

2,729) who completed surveys at three different times: between 9 and 23 days, and at 2 and 6 months after the attacks. Measures of acute stress disorder, coping style, pre-September 11 diagnoses of depression or anxiety disorders, and exposure to attack were obtained. Respondents endorsed an average of almost five positive acute stress symptoms. Posttraumatic stress symptomatology was associated with being female, marital separation, pre-September 11 depression, anxiety disorders, physical illness, severity of exposure to attacks, and early disengagement types of coping. Global distress was related to severity of loss and early coping strategies. Acute reactions were strongly predictive of later PTSD scores. Unpublished data (Silver, Holman, McIntosh, Poulin & Gil-Rivas, personal communication, October 2002) show that the Stanford Acute Stress Reaction Questionnaire (SASRQ) scales of re-experiencing and dissociation had higher positive correlations with posttraumatic stress at 2 and, especially, 6 months than hyperarousal, numbing, or functional impairment. A similar pattern was found with a different type of trauma (Harvey & Bryant, 1998).

The importance of focusing on acute posttraumatic reactions is borne out by reports that visits to a clinic for anxiety, posttraumatic, and adjustment reactions significantly increased after September 11, while those for other psychological reactions were unaffected (Galea, Resnick, & Vlahov, 2002; Hoge & Pavlin, 2002). In the last few years, following the introduction of the diagnosis of Acute Stress Disorder (ASD) into the *DSM-IV* (Cardeña, Lewis-Fernández, Beahr, Pakianathan, & Spiegel, 1996) interest in acute posttraumatic reactions, including dissociation, has increased greatly. A recent meta-analysis found dissociation around the time of trauma to be the strongest, non-demographic predictor of later PTSD (Ozer, Best, & Lipsey, 2003). Peritraumatic dissociation has also been related to maladaptive behavior at the time of trauma (Koopman, Classen, & Spiegel, 1994), and an avoidant coping style (Marmar, Weiss, Metzler, & Delucchi, 1996). Nonetheless, there is disagreement on the diagnostic value of dissociation and the best conceptualization and criteria for ASD. Additional research on the relationship between demographics, coping style, and peritraumatic dissociation is warranted (Cardeña, Butler, & Spiegel, 2003). Our study focuses on acute posttraumatic reactions to the September 11 attacks and extends previous work by analyzing acute reactions, including dissociation, in a sample containing teens, and focusing on the differential effect of coping styles and demographics.

## METHODS

### Procedure

The company Knowledge Networks (KN) administered a survey between September 20 and October 4, 2001 to gather information about people's reactions toward the September 11th terrorist attacks in New York City and Washington, DC. KN used an online research panel representative of the U.S. population. It was recruited through high quality probability sampling techniques of households through random digit dialing (RDD). Those recruited were provided with free hardware and Internet access. This methodology uses the quality standards established by the best Random Digit Dialing (RDD) surveys conducted for the Federal Government. At the time of the survey, the panel recruitment response rate was 44%. Analyses by KN show that this sample is valid and representative of the U.S. census (Knowledge Networks, 2003).

Out of all participants in KN, a sample was drawn at random from adult and adolescent active panel members. Once selected, members were notified of an important, upcoming survey. To minimize response bias, non-response adjustment was implemented using data known about those initially selected to receive the survey. For this study, non-response cells were created by cross-classifying all sample cases by age, race/ethnicity, and gender. Within each of the cross-classified cells, the initial sample weight for each case was multiplied by the non-response factor (the ratio of total assigned cases to total completed cases for that cell).

### Sample

Of the 4,250 individuals approached, 3,134 (74%) completed the questionnaire within three weeks of the attack. Our study included the adults partly analyzed in a previous study (Silver et al., 2002) plus 405 teenagers. The mean age of the sample was 43.1 ($SD = 18.7$), with a minimum age of 13 and a maximum of 101; 51.4% of the respondents were female and almost 63% were married. About 56% of the sample had some college or higher education, 61.8% reported an income of $35,000 or higher, and 69% lived in a single-family home; 73% of the sample identified themselves as white, non-Hispanic, 9% as black, 10% as Hispanic, and 7% as "other." English was the primary language of almost all participants (97%). The vast majority of respondents, 93%, were born and raised in the U.S., with 6% having been born elsewhere but moved to the U.S. more than 10 years ago, and 1% having immigrated to the U.S. in the last 10 years.

### Instruments

Demographic information was collected including gender, age, race and ethnicity, SES, religion, marital status, education, amount of September 11-related TV watching, and attitudes toward the perpetrators. Two questionnaires that are described below were administered.

*COPE Questionnaire.* The brief form of this questionnaire contains 28 items, and evaluates 14 coping styles on a 4-point scale: (1) active coping (taking action to deal with stressor), (2) planning (thinking about how to confront the stressor), (3) seeking instrumental support (seeking information on what to do), (4) seeking emotional support (getting sympathy or support), (5) religion (increased engagement in these activities), (6) positive reframing (making the best of the situation), (7) acceptance (that the stressor occurred), (8) venting (of emotions), (9) denial (trying to reject the reality of the stressor), (10) self-distraction (away from the stressor; with slight phrase changes to make items relevant for adolescents or adults), (11) behavioral disengagement (giving up with trying to cope), (12) substance use (to disengage from the stressor), (13) humor (making jokes about the stressor), and (14) self-blame (for the event) (Carver, 1997). The authors of the COPE concluded that scales 1-6 measure adaptive responses, scale 7 could be dysfunctional, whereas scales 8-10 more clearly manifest maladaptive styles. They did not offer information about the adaptive value of scales 11-14, although at face-value one would expect scales 11, 12, and 14 to be maladaptive (Carver, Scheier, & Weintraub, 1989).

*Stanford Acute Stress Reaction Questionnaire* (SASRQ). This questionnaire evaluates acute posttraumatic reactions (dissociation, re-experiencing, numbing/avoidance, hyperarousal, and functioning impairment related to the event). The SASRQ has very good reliability and validity in the adult samples in which it has been used (Cardeña, Koopman, Classen, Waelde, & Spiegel, 2000). Instead of the regular Likert scale for this measure, we used a dichotomous format (1 = not experienced, 2 = experienced), which has a published precedent (Koopman et al., 2002). To reduce the number of items for the whole survey, four questions from the questionnaire were eliminated, leaving 26 items. A few questions were slightly rephrased to make them easier to understand and applicable to teens as well as adults.

## Analyses

We measured the reliability of the modified version of the SASRQ with Cronbach's alphas and Spearman-Brown split-half analyses, and conducted bivariate analyses to evaluate the relationship between demographic, coping, behavioral and attitudinal variables, and acute distress. These were followed by stepwise multiple regressions to determine the amount of variance explained by variables significant at the bivariate level (Keppel & Zedeck, 1989). The alpha value for planned analyses was set at $p < .05$, two tailed, and Fisher's LSD correction was used for contrast comparisons. Linear and quadratic relationships were evaluated with trend analysis. Statistics were conducted using SPSS version 9.0. The study received approval from the IRB at the University of Texas-Pan American.

## RESULTS

### Psychometrics of the SASRQ

Because the psychometric properties of the SASRQ have been measured with the 30-item Likert version of the scale and with adult samples, we analyzed the version of the instrument used in this study. Internal reliability was very high for both teens and adults as measured by internal consistency (alphas = .88, .87, respectively) and split-half correlations ($rs$ = .82, .79, respectively). Construct and convergent validity were supported by data presented in the following section, which shows, for instance, that greater exposure (i.e., living in NYC) and female gender were related to distress, as found in studies reviewed earlier.

### Demographic Variables and Attitudes

Every respondent endorsed at least one SASRQ item. The four most common items were: feeling on edge ($M = 1.40$, $SD = .49$), a sense of timelessness ($M = 1.34$, $SD = .47$), mind going blank ($M = 1.34$, $SD = .47$), and restlessness ($M = 1.33$, $SD = .47$). As Table 1 shows, women, foreign born, divorced or never married (as compared to married), and young adults (18-44) reported more distress. Neither level of income, ethnicity, education, or religion were associated with acute distress. Multivariate analysis showed that, in order of decreasing variance explained, TV watching, gender, age, and place of birth remained significant. Marital status was no longer significant (Table 2).

## TABLE 1. ANOVA for SASRQ scores by demographics

| Variable | M (SD) | F | Sig. | Eta sq. |
|---|---|---|---|---|
| TV Watched | | 43.3 | < 0.001 | 0.04 |
| < 1 Hr./day | 29.75 (4.64)* | | | |
| 1-3 Hrs./day | 30.64 (4.79)* | | | |
| 4-6 Hrs./day | 31.66 (4.87)* | | | |
| > 6 Hrs./day | 33.02 (5.65)* | | | |
| Gender | | 92.1 | < 0.001 | 0.029 |
| Male | 30.18 (4.69) | | | |
| Female | 31.94 (5.45) | | | |
| Born | | 182 | 0.001 | 0.005 |
| U.S. Born | 31.02 (5.06)** | | | |
| Moved to U.S. > 10 yrs | 32.29 (5.47)** | | | |
| Moved to U.S. < 10 yrs | 32.65 (5.62)** | | | |
| Age | | 130 | < 0.001 | 0.01 |
| 13-17 | 30.51 (5.12) | | | |
| 18-24 | 31.72 (5.94)[a] | | | |
| 25-34 | 31.86 (5.63)[b] | | | |
| 35-44 | 31.53 (5.08)[c] | | | |
| 45-54 | 30.95 (5.02) | | | |
| 55-64 | 30.75 (4.80) | | | |
| 65-74 | 30.41 (4.71) | | | |
| 75+ | 30.34 (4.82) | | | |
| Marital Status | | 2.83 | 0.023 | 0.004 |
| Married | 30.98 (5.04)[d] | | | |
| Never Married | 31.61 (5.64) | | | |
| Divorced | 31.66 (5.15) | | | |
| Widowed | 30.58 (4.34)[e] | | | |
| Separated | 31.93 (6.25) | | | |

Note: Level of income, ethnicity, religion and level of education were not significantly related to acute distress.
*$p < .001$ for all contrasts
**$p < .05$ for all contrasts
[a]$p < .05$ or less for contrasts with 13-17, 55-64, 65-74, and 75+
[b]$p < .05$ or less for contrasts with 13-17, 45-54, 55-64, 65-74, and 75+
[c]$p < .05$ or less for contrasts with 13-17, 55-64, 65-74, 75+
[d]$p < .05$ for contrasts with never married and divorced
[e]$p < .05$ for contrast with never married

TABLE 2. Stepwise regression analyses for demographic variables predicting SASRQ scores

| | B (SE) | Beta | Adj. R sq. |
|---|---|---|---|
| Step 1 | | | .039* |
| TV watching | 1.10 (.10) | .198 | |
| Step 2 | | | .063* |
| TV watching | .97 (.10) | .175 | |
| Gender | 1.59 (.19) | .158 | |
| Step 3 | | | .078* |
| TV watching | 1.03 (.10) | .187 | |
| Gender | 1.60 (.19) | .159 | |
| Age | −.38 (.05) | −.124 | |
| Step 4 | | | .082* |
| TV watching | 1.03 (.10) | .187 | |
| Gender | 1.60 (.19) | .159 | |
| Age | −.36 (.05) | −.120 | |
| Place of birth | .983 (.27) | .066 | |

*$p < .001$

Increased hours of TV watching were linearly associated with greater distress ($F = 803.39$, $df = 1, 3104$, $p < .001$). The effect of age on SASRQ scores was quadratic or curvilinear ($F = 1,150.57$, $df = 1, 1150$, $p < .001$), showing that distress levels were lower for those younger and older than middle-range adults (see Figure 1).

When looking at location, the only region that showed greater distress than the rest of the nation was New York City ($M = 34.07$, $SD = 5.56$ vs. $M = 31.03$, $SD = 5.17$; $F = 28.5$, $df = 1, 2764$, $p < .001$, eta sq. = .01), which suffered the most severe attack. Analyses of the adolescent sub-sample by itself showed that being female and TV watching remained significantly related to distress, but immigration did not ($F = 8.6$, $df = 1, 402$, $p = .003$; $F = 4.5$, $df = 3, 396$, $p = .004$; $F = 0.1$, $df = 2, 397$, $p = .89$, respectively). Teens did not show greater dissociation than any other group when that subscale of the SASRQ was evaluated ($p > .1$ for all comparisons), but females reporter greater dissociation than males ($M = 12.29$, $SD = 2.33$ vs. $M = 11.65$, $SD = 2.06$, $F = 65.32$, $df = 1, 3120$, $p < .001$).

FIGURE 1. SASRQ scores by age

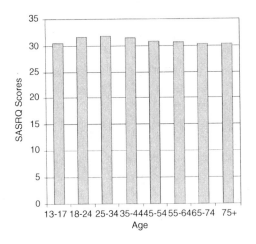

Three of the four items measuring aggression toward the perpetrators ("I felt a need to punish those responsible for the terrorist attacks," "I felt a desire to hurt the people who did this," and "We need to wipe out those responsible for these attacks") had very small but significant positive correlations with the SASRQ ($r = .09$ being the largest, $p < .01$ for all analyses); war as the only possible response to the attack was unrelated. These four items had significant but small positive correlations with TV watching ($r = .13$ being the largest, $p < .001$ for all analyses).

## Coping

The most commonly endorsed coping styles were acceptance ($M = 6.59, SD = 1.45$), turning to religion ($M = 5.20, SD = 2.21$), and venting ($M = 4.49, SD = 1.69$). All but one of the scales (humor) and the SASRQ had significant but small correlations (average $r = .19$; $p < .001$ for all analyses; all correlations were positive except for "acceptance," $r = -.13$).

Multiple regression revealed that all of the COPE subscales significant at the bivariate level except for "active coping" and "positive reframing" continued to predict distress when controlling for the effects of the other subscales. Together they accounted for almost 30% of the variance in SASRQ scores. The seeking emotional support, self-blame, denial, venting, and behavioral disengagement scales explained most of the variance. A similar analysis just for the teens showed a very similar pattern of results, the only difference being that self-distraction was among the five most common coping styles used by teens, but venting was not.

A multivariate analysis that included the COPE and demographic variables previously identified as significant predictors of SASRQ scores (seeking emotional support, self-blaming, denial, venting, behavioral disengagement, TV watching, self-distraction, acceptance, planning, gender, substance use, instrumental support, self-distraction, age, turning to religion, and place of birth) resulted in place of birth no longer being significant. Including demographic variables increased the variance explained by coping only by about 4%; these variables, except for TV watching, explained less variance than any of the coping scales.

In order of decreasing magnitude, venting, planning, seeking emotional support, turning to religion, self-distraction (for adults), denial, active coping, seeking instrumental support, and humor had significant, but small (highest $r = .18$; $p < .001$ for all analyses) correlations with TV watching, all of them positive except for self-distraction and humor. Multiple comparisons revealed that participants 13-24 years of age experienced greater self-distraction than other age categories; they also sought out more instrumental support, and exhibited greater behavioral disengagement than middle-aged respondents. This group (13-24) also vented, planned and accepted what had happened less than older individuals ($p < .01$ for all analyses). Women scored higher than men on self-distraction, active coping, denial, seeking emotional support, behavioral disengagement, venting, positive reframing, and turning to religion; males scored higher on substance abuse, planning, humor, and acceptance ($p < .01$ for all analyses).

## DISCUSSION

Acute distress was related to being a New York resident, being female, a young adult, having immigrated to the U.S., and watching TV. New York area residents suffered the most severe and lingering attacks, so their greater distress confirms the association between exposure and greater distress (Fullerton et al., 2001; Galea et al., 2002; Schlenger et al., 2002; Schuster et al., 2001). Previous research has shown that being female is related to posttraumatic distress, although inconsistently (Brewin, Andrews, & Valentine, 2000). There is some evidence that females exhibit greater peritraumatic dissociation than males (Cardeña et al., 2003), as we found, and that this type of reaction may be a greater risk factor of later PTSD for females than for males (Fullerton et al., 2001). This difference may be explained by a greater tendency by women to report distress, to perceive life events as more distressing (Caballo & Cardeña, 1997), and/or by a greater use of some dysfunctional forms of coping (Carver et al., 1989). In our data the gender effect disappeared when controlling for coping styles. Females, as compared with males, reported more dysfunctional coping styles, two of which, seeking self-support and venting, were among the top styles accounting for SASRQ variance. Maladaptive coping may serve as a mediating variable for acute distress, since coping to a specific situation is moderately correlated with dispositional forms of coping (Carver et al., 1989).

Although marital status was marginally related to distress in bivariate analyses, as found in other studies (Brewin et al., 2000), the relationship vanished when controlling for other demographics, as was also true in research with a less representative sample (Galea et al., 2002). We found that young adults were most affected by the events of 9/11, as did Schlenger et al. (2002), but because we also included teenagers in our survey we found the relationship between acute distress and age to be curvilinear. Contrary to studies measuring trait dissociation (Vanderlinden, Van der Hart & Varga, 1996), teens did not show greater state dissociation than adults. The fact that teens mentioned less distress than young adults could be explained by the fact that the SASRQ had not been previously validated with that age group, but our analyses run counter to that conclusion. A more likely explanation is that young adults were more distressed because of their greater identification with the victims of the attacks, which seemed to be mostly young adults; similarity with trauma victims is related to posttraumatic reactions (Dixon, Rehling, & Schiwach, 1993). Contrary to previous studies (Galea et al., 2002; Schuster et al., 2001), there was no effect for ethnicity, perhaps because of the more representative nature of our sample, including various socioeconomic levels (see also Zatzick, Marmar, Weiss, & Metzler, 1994). Our findings suggest that those who immigrated into the U.S. had higher distress, perhaps because of less social support (Brewin et al., 2000), or the effect of immigration.

Of all of the demographic and related variables, TV watching explained the most variance in post-attack distress. A study of children following the Oklahoma City bombing reported that TV viewing was associated with greater distress (Pfefferbaum et al., 2001). Other studies extended this finding to adults (Schlenger et al., 2002; Schuster et al., 2001; Silver et al., 2002) while we found this effect among teens.

Schlenger et al. (2002) proposed that TV watching may be considered a form of coping; however, the small correlations we found between coping styles and TV watching does not support this interpretation. It is more likely that distress primed viewers to pay particular attention to threatening information, and that continued exposure to such information increased distress in a circular fashion (McNaughton-Cassill & Smith, 2002). Instead of the thoughtful elaboration that may be necessary for relief of traumatic memories (Cardeña, Maldonado, Van der Hart, & Spiegel, 2000; Pennebaker, 1997), TV coverage of the attack was dominated by sensational and gruesome imagery, perhaps reactivating anxiety and fear without providing ways to reprocess them. The relationship between aggression toward the perpetrators and TV watching might be partly explained by the distress generated by watching the news, but the very small correlations make any hypothesis highly tentative.

Predictably, the more distress people had, the more they reported using coping strategies. The two exceptions were "humor" (an unlikely form of coping given the severity of the attacks) and "acceptance" (greater acceptance was related to less distress). We found that coping strategies were more strongly associated with acute distress than demographic variables, as did other samples that did not include teens (Silver et al., 2002; Harvey & Bryant, 1998). Four of the five coping style that explained most of the variance in our data (self-blame, denial, venting, and behavioral disengagement) have been considered maladaptive in previous research with less severe stressors (Carver, 1997), and there is evidence that initial disengagement and self-blame predict later PTSD (Mellman, Bustamante, Fins, & Esposito, 2001). Our data suggest that adaptive coping may not account for as much variance in distress when dealing with traumatic events as defensive and maladaptive strategies, and underline the importance of coping strategies in long-term posttraumatic reactions (Gibbs, 1989; Spiegel, 2002). The data that younger respondents endorsed more self-distraction and behavioral disengagement, but less planning and acceptance support the idea that adaptive coping tends not to be manifested until late adulthood (Blanchard-Fields & Irion, 1988).

Because process and dispositional variables seem to be better predictors of posttraumatic distress than demographics, prevention and intervention strategies should seek to identify and reduce maladaptive strategies, especially among groups that are likely to be more affected either because of exposure and/or identification with the victims. Although causality cannot be inferred from our data, our results suggest that watching many hours of TV coverage of traumatic events may exacerbate distress.

This study has strengths and limitations. The representative nationwide sample and data collection shortly after the attacks provide stronger generalizability than is found in most trauma studies, and this study may be the first one to include responses by adolescents to 9/11. We employed validated instruments and analyzed various potential contributing factors to acute posttraumatic distress. Limitations of the study include the lack of pre-event measures, which may explain a substantial amount of variance (Silver et al., 2002), its cross-sectional nature, and the inability to determine to what extent SASRQ scores translate to clinical impairment. Yet, this study may be unique in its analysis of reactions to 9/11 in a sample containing adolescents and measuring the differential contribution of demographics and coping styles.

# REFERENCES

Blanchard-Fields, F., & Irion, J.C. (1988). Coping strategies from the perspective of two developmental markers: Age and social reasoning. *Journal of Genetic Psychology, 149*, 141-151.

Brewin, C., Andrews, B., & Valentine, J.D. (2000). Meta-analysis of risk factors for posttraumatic stress disorder in trauma-exposed adults. *Journal of Consulting and Clinical Psychology, 68*, 748-766.

Caballo, V.E., & Cardeña, E. (1997). Sex differences in the perception of stressful life events: Some implications for the Axis IV of DSM-IV. *Journal of Personality and Individual Differences, 23*, 353-359.

Cardeña, E., Butler, L.D., & Spiegel, D. (2003). Disorders of extreme stress. In T.A. Widiger (Ed.), *Comprehensive handbook of psychology* (pp. 229-249). New York, NY: John Wiley.

Cardeña, E., Koopman, C., Classen, C., Waelde, L. & Spiegel, D. (2000). Psychometric properties of the Stanford Acute Stress Reaction Questionnaire (SASRQ): A valid and reliable measure of acute stress reactions. *Journal of Traumatic Stress, 13*, 719-734.

Cardeña, E., Lewis-Fernández, R., Beahr, D., Pakianathan, I., & Spiegel, D. (1996). Dissociative disorders. In T.A. Widiger, A.J. Frances, H.J. Pincus, R. Ross, M.B. First, & W.W. Davis (Eds.), *Sourcebook for the DSM-IV. Vol. II.* (pp. 973-1005). Washington, DC: American Psychiatric Press.

Cardeña, E., Maldonado, J., Van der Hart, O., & Spiegel, D. (2000). Hypnosis. In E. Foa, T. Keane, & M. Friedman (Eds.), *Effective treatments for PTSD* (pp. 407-440). New York, NY: Guilford Press.

Carver, C.S. (1997). You want to measure coping but your protocol's too long: Consider the Brief COPE. *International Journal of Behavioral Medicine, 4*, 92-100.

Carver, C. S., Scheier, M.F., & Weintraub, J.K. (1989). Assessing coping strategies: A theoretically based approach. *Journal of Personality and Social Psychology, 56,* 267-283.

Dixon, P., Rehling, G., & Shiwach, R. (1993). Peripheral victims of the Herald of Free Enterprise disaster. *British Journal of Medical Psychology, 66,* 193-202.

Fullerton, C.S., Ursano, R.J., Epstein, R.S., Crowley, B., Vance, K., Kao, T.C., Dougall, A, & Baum, A. (2001). Gender differences in posttraumatic stress disorder after motor vehicle accidents. *American Journal of Psychiatry, 158,* 1486-1491.

Galea, S., Ahern, J., Resnick, H., Kilpatrick, D., Bucuvalas, M., Gold, J., & Vlahov, D. (2002). Psychological sequelae of the September 11 terrorist attacks in New York City. *New England Journal of Medicine, 346,* 982-987.

Galea, S., Resnick, H., & Vlahov, D. (2002). Psychological sequelae of September 11. *New England Journal of Medicine, 347,* 444-445.

Gibbs, M.S. (1989). Factors in the victim that mediate between disaster and psychopathology: A review. *Journal of Traumatic Stress, 2,* 489-514.

Harvey, A.G., & Bryant, R.A. (1998). Relationship of acute stress disorder and posttraumatic stress disorder following motor vehicle accidents. *Journal of Consulting Clinical Psychology, 66,* 507-512.

Hoge, C.W., & Pavlin, J.A. (2002). Psychological sequelae of September 11. *New England Journal of Medicine, 347,* 443.

Keppel, G., & Zedeck, S. (1989). *Data analysis for research designs.* New York, NY: Freeman.

Koopman, C., Classen, C., & Spiegel, D. (1994). Predictors of posttraumatic stress symptoms among survivors of the Oakland/Berkeley, Calif., firestorm. *American Journal of Psychiatry, 151,* 888-894.

Koopman, C., Gore-Felton, C., Azimi, N., O'Shea, K., Ashton, E., Power, R., De Maria, S., Israelski, D., & Spiegel, D. (2002). Acute stress reactions to life events among women and men living with HIV/AIDS. *International Journal of Psychiatry and Medicine, 32,* 361-378.

Knowledge Networks. (2003, May). *Validity of the survey of health and Internet and Knowledge Network's panel and sampling.* Retrieved December 9, 2003, from http://www.herc.research.med.va.gov/SHI%20appendix.pdf

Marmar, C.R., Weiss, D.S., Metzler, T.J., & Delucchi, K. (1996). Characteristics of emergency services personnel related to peritraumatic dissociation during critical incident exposure. *American Journal of Psychiatry, 153,* 94-102.

McNaughton-Cassill, M.E., & Smith, T. My world is OK, but yours is not: Television news, the optimism gap, and stress. *Stress and Health, 18,* 27-33.

Mellman, T.A., David, D., Bustamante, V., Fins, A.I., & Esposito, K. (2001). Predictors of post-traumatic stress disorder following severe injury. *Depression & Anxiety, 14,* 226-231.

North, C., & Pfefferbaum, B. (2002). Research on the mental health effects of terrorism. *Journal of the American Medical Association, 288,* 633-636.

Ozer, E., Best, S., & Lipsey, T. (2003). Predictors of posttraumatic stress disorder-symptoms in adults: A meta-analysis. *Psychological Bulletin, 129,* 52-73.

Pennebaker, J. (1997). *Opening up.* New York, NY: Guilford.

Pfefferbaum, B., Nixon, S.J., Tivis, R.D., Doughty, D.E., Pynoos, R.S., Gurwitch, R.H., & Foy, D.W. (2001). Television exposure in children after a terrorist incident. *Psychiatry, 64,* 202-211.

Schlenger, W.E., Caddell, J.M., Ebert, L., Jordan, B.K., Rourke, K.M., Wilson, D., Thalji, L., Dennis, J.M., Fairbank, J.A., & Kulka, R.A. (2002). Psychological reactions to terrorist attacks. Findings from the national study of Americans' reactions to September 11. *Journal of the American Medical Association, 288,* 581-588.

Schuster, M.A., Stein, B.D., Jaycox, L.H., Collins, R.L., Marshall, G.N., Elliot, M.N., Zhou, A. J., Kanouse, D.E., Morrison. J.L., & Berry, S.H. (2001). A national survey of stress reactions after the September 11, 2001, terrorist attacks. *New England Journal of Medicine, 345,* 1507-1512.

Silver, R.C., Holman, A., McIntosh, D.N., Pouli, M., Gil-Rivas, V. (2002). Nationwide longitudinal study of psychological responses to September 11. *Journal of American Medical Association, 228,* 1235-1244.

Spiegel, D. (2002). Acute stress symptoms and coping after the terrorist attacks: Internet survey results. Paper presented at the American Psychological Annual Convention, Chicago, IL.

Vanderlinden, J, Van der Hart, O., & Varga, K. (1996). European studies of Dissociation. In L. Michelson & W.J. Ray (Eds.), *Handbook of dissociation: Theoretical, empirical, and clinical perspectives* (pp. 25-49). New York, NY: Plenum Press.

Zatzick, D.F., Marmar, C.R., Weiss, D.S., & Metzler, T. (1994). Does trauma-linked dissociation vary across ethnic groups? *Journal of Nervous & Mental Disease, 182,* 576-582.

# Risk Factors for Psychological Adjustment Following Residential Fire: The Role of Avoidant Coping

Russell T. Jones, PhD
Thomas H. Ollendick, PhD

**SUMMARY.** Although a growing number of investigations have targeted technological and natural disasters involving children and adolescents (e.g., kidnappings, shootings, accidents, wars, fires, hurricanes), little is known about the influence of specific risk factors on functioning post-disaster. A number of basic questions are yet to be fully addressed, including: How do children and adolescents cope with technological and natural disasters? What are the most salient risk factors for children and adolescents, prior to, during, and following disasters? How do these risk factors interact in predicting psychological adjustment? And what is the relative role of risk factors on psychological adjustment over time? In fact, these and related questions hold the potential

Russell T. Jones and Thomas H. Ollendick are affiliated with the Department of Psychology, Virginia Polytechnic Institute and State University, Blacksburg, VA.

Address correspondence to: Russell T. Jones, PhD, Professor of Psychology, Virginia Polytechnic Institute and State University, Department of Psychology, 5088 Derring Hall, Blacksburg, VA 24061-0436 (E-mail: rtjones@vt.edu).

This project was funded in part from a NIMH grant, number 5R01 MH049147-04–Children's Reactions to Residential Fires, as well as a grant from the Georgia Firefighters Burn Foundation, number 433849.

[Haworth co-indexing entry note]: "Risk Factors for Psychological Adjustment Following Residential Fire: The Role of Avoidant Coping" Jones, Russell T., and Thomas H. Ollendick. Co-published simultaneously in *Journal of Trauma & Dissociation* (The Haworth Medical Press, an imprint of The Haworth Press, Inc.) Vol. 6, No. 2, 2005, pp. 85-99; and: *Acute Reactions to Trauma and Psychotherapy: A Multidisciplinary and International Perspective* (ed: Etzel Cardeña, and Kristin Croyle) The Haworth Medical Press, an imprint of The Haworth Press, Inc., 2005, pp. 85-99. Single or multiple copies of this article are available for a fee from The Haworth Document Delivery Service [1-800-HAWORTH, 9:00 a.m. - 5:00 p.m. (EST). E-mail address: docdelivery@haworthpress.com].

Available online at http://www.haworthpress.com/web/JTD
© 2005 by The Haworth Press, Inc. All rights reserved.
doi:10.1300/J229v06n02_08

to move this important area of inquiry forward in a variety of meaningful ways. *[Article copies available for a fee from The Haworth Document Delivery Service: 1-800-HAWORTH. E-mail address: <docdelivery@haworthpress.com> Website: <http://www.HaworthPress.com> © 2005 by The Haworth Press, Inc. All rights reserved.]*

**KEYWORDS.** Coping, children, adolescents, disaster, fire

The purpose of this brief paper is to highlight major risk factors that have been explored in the child and adolescent disaster literature. Concerted attention is given to avoidance coping as a risk factor and its potential implications on a young person's functioning following a disaster. Examples from the extant literature as well as our NIMH-funded grant designed to assess the impact of residential fire on children and adolescents will be presented. Several recommendations for future research efforts will also be proffered.

As frequently noted in the clinical child and pediatric psychology literature, there are few agreed-upon risk factors associated with technological and natural disasters. However, those factors most frequently cited can be organized temporally as follows: pre-trauma, during-trauma, and post-trauma. More specifically, in the pre-trauma category, the following factors are often cited: developmental level, gender, cultural and ethnicity factors, pre-morbid functioning, family functioning, pre-trauma schemas, risk for exposure, and a host of person-related factors (e.g., locus of control, personal efficacy, anxiety, self-esteem, self-worth). During-trauma factors include: characteristics of the stressor itself, exposure (e.g., loss, life threat), major life events, social support, and parental functioning. Finally, during the post-trauma phase, major life events, social support, coping styles, self-efficacy, and parental functioning are typically specified as risk factors (see Saigh & Bremner, 1999; and Pfefferbaum, 1997; for reviews). Unfortunately, no systematic effort has been undertaken to more precisely place each of these factors into one of the three phases of the disaster event. Nor has anyone specified the degree to which each factor may be present across all three phases of the disaster experience. Nonetheless, a considerable amount of effort has been put into the study of several of these factors.

In our program of research aimed at the assessment and treatment of the psychosocial consequences of fire we have been able to examine the role of several of these risk factors. More specifically, we have studied the influence of gender, race, socio-economic status, social support, parent's reactions and coping on children and adolescents' functioning following residential fire (see Jones & Ollendick, 2002, for a review).

Our model consists of four primary components: (1) characteristics of the stressor, (2) characteristics of the children, (3) characteristics of the environment, and (4) the cognitive processing of the fire experience by the children, adolescents, and their families. Within the context of this model, we have been able to study systematically the separate and interactive impact of these factors following the trauma over time (six months and one year later).

In spite of the fact that there is little consensus on how to best conceptualize or measure coping (Skinner, Edge, Altman, & Sherwood, 2003), it has been viewed as a major determinant of adjustment in a variety of stressful situations. Further study of the role of different coping strategies in the context of disasters (i.e., prior to, during, after) may be quite useful and informative. More specifically, avoidant coping may be a particularly important risk factor to study in that avoidance itself is a core symptom of posttraumatic stress disorder and specific phobias associated with the traumatic event. Moreover, a variety of avoidance-type behaviors have been shown to occur during and following traumatic events.

Within the clinical child area, coping has been conceptualized as both a mediator (Thompson, Kronenberger, Johnson, & Whiting, 1989) and a moderator (Davies & Cummings, 1995) of the effects of trauma. (See Holmbeck, 1997 for an excellent discussion concerning the appropriateness and distinction between such conceptualizations.) Briefly, mediation tests the role of an independent variable (e.g., social support) that might explain "why" a relationship exits between the predictor (e.g., resource loss) and the criterion (e.g., coping strategies) variables. Conversely, moderation specifies "when" or "under what conditions" a relationship exists between the independent variable (e.g., social support) and the predictor (i.e., resource loss) and criterion (i.e., coping strategies) variables. Whether best conceptualized as a mediator or a moderator, avoidant coping is frequently found to be a significant risk factor. A risk factor has been defined as "any condition or circumstance that increases the likelihood that psychopathology will develop" (Wenar & Kerig, 2000, p. 20). Avoidant coping in specific contexts clearly meets this definition.

Indeed, avoidant coping has been shown to increase the likelihood of distress across several domains. In the context of disaster situations avoidant coping style may enhance the level of distress. That is, as individuals engage in maladaptive avoidance coping strategies, they are more likely to experience undesired outcomes. Although there may be instances in which avoidance strategies are adaptive and protect the in-

88 Acute Reactions to Trauma and Psychotherapy

dividual (e.g., immediately following the event), the focal point of this discussion will be on those situations where such forms of coping are maladaptive and do not lead to reductions in levels of distress, but rather to heightened levels of distress.

For example, in their work assessing children following parental divorce, Sandler, Tein, and West (1994) found avoidant coping to be significantly and positively related to child depression, anxiety, and conduct problems. Additionally, they reported that avoidant coping appeared to serve a mediational role in the relationship between stress and psychological symptomatology: that is, stress led to the use of avoidant coping strategies which in turn led to maladaptive outcomes. They also suggested that avoidant coping served to make the child or adolescent more aware of their distress and to actually potentiate it. In a related investigation with children of divorced parents, avoidance coping was also found to be positively related to depression and conduct problems, and negatively related to self-esteem (Ayers, Sandler, West, & Roosa, 1996).

In the literature examining parental behavior and family environment, several investigations have documented the relation between avoidant coping and distress. For example, in studying the relations among parental chronic illness, internalizing problems, family processes, and avoidant coping, Steele, Forehand, and Armistead (1997) found that severity of father's illness, negative parent-child relations, and avoidant coping strategies were significantly related with one another and led to negative outcomes. Similarly, children whose parents modeled low levels of cognitive restructuring in times of distress have also been reported to engage in avoidant coping (Kliewer & Lewis, 1995), whereas children with parents who were more responsive were more likely to engage in problem-focused coping (McKernon et al., 2001).

Furthermore, examples of the negative impact of avoidance coping may be gleaned from the emerging coping efficacy literature. Defined as a child or adolescent's subjective appraisal of their ability to cope with the demands of a stressful or traumatic situation (Bandura, 1986), coping efficacy has been hypothesized to impact positively upon behavior outcomes (Bandura, 1997). That is, when coping efficacy beliefs are high, one's behavior may be aimed at actively rectifying pressing environmental and emotional demands. Conversely, when coping efficacy is low, greater energy is likely to be directed toward avoidant coping strategies. Although published reports documenting the role of self-efficacy with children in disaster situations are yet to appear, among adults in a post-disaster situation a negative relationship between coping self-efficacy and avoidant coping has been reported (Benight et al., 1998).

In our own work, we have identified instances where avoidant coping has operated as a risk factor for fear associated with traumatic situations. In a recent paper we examined the roles of negative life events, attributional styles, and avoidant coping strategies in the prediction of fear (Ollendick, Langley, Jones, & Kephart, 2001). Briefly, 46 children and adolescents enrolled in our residential fire project (see Jones & Ollendick, 2002) participated. Families were compensated $75 for their participation. The sample consisted of 56.5% females, with a mean age of 11 years 10 months (range 8 years to 16 years). The sample was primarily Caucasians (52.2%) and African Americans (43.5%). Hispanic (2.2%) and Biracial youth (2.2%) were represented in smaller proportions. With respect to family structure, 45% of the participants lived in single parent families (mother), 25% in divorced but re-married families, and 30% in two-parent families. The average level of maternal education was at the high school level. When examining this sample in categories of high or low levels of education, 41.3% reported low parental education levels (7th grade to high school graduate), and 58.7% reported high levels (some college to graduate degree). Each child was interviewed individually within approximately three months following the fire.

Several measures were administered as part of a larger interview conducted in the participants' homes, neighborhood churches, libraries, or Red Cross offices by advanced graduate clinicians. The entire interview took approximately three hours to complete. Instruments included The Life Events Checklist, KASTAN Children's Attributional Style Questionnaire-Revised, The How I Coped Under Pressure Scale, and the Revised Fear Survey Schedule for Children. Negative life events were assessed with the Life Events Checklist (LEC; Johnson & McCutcheon, 1980), a 46-item child and adolescent self-report measure, utilized to assess the number and perceived impact of stressful life events that occurred in the participant's life in the past year. Each event is classified as "bad" or "good" and then its impact is rated on a scale from 0 to 3 (0 = no effect, and 3 = great effect). The scale yields positive life events and negative life events score. Acceptable validity (Johnson & McCutcheon, 1980) and reliability for positive, negative, and total life events on the LEC have been reported (Brand & Johnson, 1982). Representative items include "Mother or father lost job," "Increased absence of parents from the home" and "Moving to a new home."

The KASTAN Children's Attributional Style Questionnaire-Revised (KASTAN-R-CASQ; Kaslow, Tanenbaum, & Seligman, 1978) was used in this study to assess attributional style for children and adolescents. The CASQ is a 48-item forced choice instrument measuring causal attributions to an equal number of positive and negative hypothetical situations. The scale yields a negative, a positive and a composite score as well as a total difference score (positive-negative composites). For purposes of the current analyses, difference scores were employed. Moderate reliability estimates have been reported for this measure in previous studies ($\alpha$'s ranging from .42 to .67).

How I Coped Under Pressure Scale (HICUPS; Ayers et al., 1996) is a 45-item self-report checklist that asks children and adolescents to indicate how often they have engaged each of a list of coping strategies based on a 4-point Likert scale (1 = not at all, 2 = a little, 3 = somewhat, 4 = a lot) in coping with a single specified incident. Items for this scale were created to reflect the ten distinct categories, grouped into four factors (Active coping, Distraction strategies, Avoidance, and Support seeking). These factors were identified by Ayers et al. (1996), and Sandler et al. (1994) through a content analysis of children's coping responses. The scale was found to demonstrate acceptable internal consistencies, as measured by coefficient alpha, ranging from .57 to .74 for the ten subscales. Participants in this study were asked to complete the questionnaire with reference to the strategies they utilized to cope with the residential fire.

Lastly, the Revised Fear Survey Schedule for Children (FSSC-R; Ollendick, 1983) was used to assess level of fear. The FSSC-R is a fear inventory consisting of 80 items, devised to assess the frequency, intensity, and content of children's fears. Level of fear is self-rated on a scale of 1 to 3 (1 = none, 2 = some, and 3 = a lot) for each of the 80 items. In addition to a total score, the FSSC-R yields five subscales, derived from factor analyses: Fear of the Unknown, Fear of Minor Injury and Small Animals, Fear of Death and Danger, Medical Fears, and Fear of Failure and Criticism. These factors have been shown to have satisfactory internal consistency and to be stable across cultures. Likewise, the FSSC-R has been shown to have acceptable test-retest reliability and validity estimates.

Avoidant coping as defined by Ayers et al. (1996) consists of behavioral strategies to evade the stressor or reminders of the stressor, repress thoughts about it, or engage in wishful thinking. Results of this study showed negative life events, negative attributional styles, and avoidant coping predicted heightened levels of fear.

Although negative life events were associated with the level of fear for children from families with low levels of maternal education, avoidant coping and negative attributional styles predicted fear in those individuals whose mother had high levels of education. The zero-order correlations reported in Tables 1 and 2 depict these relations. We found the moderating role of maternal education to be intriguing. Specifically, level of maternal education served a protective function; that is, a high level of education lessened the impact of negative life events including residential fire. We speculated that because of their parent's greater access to resources (e.g., finances, support), the relationship between the fire and fear was not significant in these children. However, because they may have been less adept at coping with infrequently occurring negative life events, they engaged in greater levels of avoidant coping that, in turn, was related to heightened fear levels.

With respect to avoidant coping among children whose parents possessed low levels of education, we reasoned that cognitive processes including negative attributional styles might have diminished the use of avoidant coping. That is, because of the chronicity and persistence of negative life events stemming from factors including poverty, and low socio-economic status, children may have adopted this negative attributional style. Additionally however, given the immediate threat to well-being and safety resulting from the loss of possessions and the possibility of relocation, these children may have felt that avoidant coping would serve no functional role in this situation. In fact, it may have been the case that many of these children felt that they had to be actively involved in the restorative process. They may have reasoned that "if things are going to be restored, I must restore them." We hope to address each of these lines of reasoning in future investigations.

TABLE 1. Zero-Order Correlations for Low Maternal Education Between Fear (FSSC-R), Negative Life Events (NLE-I), Attributional Style (CASQ), and Avoidant Coping (AVC)

| Variable/Measure | FSSC-R | NLE-I | CASQ |
|---|---|---|---|
| NLE-I | .45** | | |
| CASQ | −.27 | −.29* | |
| AVC | .10 | .09 | .02 |

Note: $N = 42$; $*p < .10$, $**p < .01$

TABLE 2. Zero-Order Correlations for High Maternal Education Between Fear (FSSC-R), Negative Life Events (NLE-I), Attributional Style (CASQ), and Avoidant Coping (AVC)

| Variable/Measure | FSSC-R | NLE-I | CASQ |
|---|---|---|---|
| NLE-I | .10 | | |
| CASQ | −.24 | −.01 | |
| AVC | .41*** | −.21 | .12 |

*Note: N = 57; ***p < .001*

In a second investigation aimed at assessing predictors of coping (Jones, Wang, & Ollendick, in preparation), we addressed the question: "What influences children's choice of coping strategies?" In the context of the previously mentioned grant, 92 children and adolescents served as participants. We examined relative impact of dispositional variables (i.e., demographic characteristics, self-worth) and situational variables including, resource loss, negative life events, social support, and coping efficacy on the use of coping strategies (i.e., active, avoidance, distraction, social support seeking) in children and adolescents three months following residential fire. In addition to the Educational Factor classification of Hollingshead's (1975) Index of Social Status, the How I Coped Under Pressure Scale (HICUPS; Ayers et al., 1996) and the Life Events Checklist (LEC; Johnson & McCutcheon, 1980) were employed in the current investigation. For purposes of this investigation, the impact of negative life events perceived as *not* related to the fire was used.

Loss was measured through a modified version of Freedy's Resource Loss Scale (Freedy, Shaw, Jarrell, & Masters, 1992) that assesses four dimensions of loss: object loss (i.e., tangible possessions lost due to the fire such as clothing and toys), energy loss (e.g., free time), condition loss (e.g., a good relationship with my parents), and personal characteristics loss (e.g., sense of humor). Children first respond "yes" or "no" to whether or not they experienced any loss of each item. If they answer "yes" to an item, they are further asked to indicate the extent of the loss on a 3-point scale (1 = a little, 2 = some, 3 = a lot). The sum of the impact of loss yields the total loss score. All questions were asked in reference to the fire. The children provided a rich array of comments about specific losses and how those losses affected their lives.

The Child's Subjective Appraisals of family, teacher, and peer support (APP; Dubow & Ullman, 1989) is a 9-item assessment tool that contains items with the highest factor loadings from an original 41-item version designed to measure children's subjective appraisals of family, teacher, and peer social support. Participants are asked to respond to questions using a 5-point Likert scale. Lower scores indicated that the participant perceived a low level of availability of support from family, teachers, or peers, while higher scores suggested that the participant perceived a high level of availability of support from these individuals. Internal consistency has been reported as .88, while test-retest reliability for a three to four week period has been found to be .75 (Dubow & Ullman, 1989). In order to obtain a measure of fire-related social support for this investigation, three newly devised items were added to this instrument. The format of these items was consistent with the wording of the same of the three additional items used (e.g., "Some kids feel that they are free to talk with their family about a number of things, but other kids don't feel this way. Do you feel that you are able to talk with your teachers about the fire?").

The Self-Perception Profile for Children (SPPC; Harter, 1985) is a 36-item scale devised to measure children's self-competence in a number of domains as well as global perceptions of self-esteem. Each item contains two statements that are antithetical to each other (e.g., "Some kids like the kind of person they are, BUT Other kids wish that they were different"). Each child chooses one of the statements and then rates it as really true or sort-of true. While this scale provides a score for six subscales (i.e., scholastic competence, social acceptance, athletic competence, physical appearance, behavioral conduct, and global self-worth), only the global self-worth (GSW) subscale was used in the present investigation. This subscale contains six items with half the items reverse-worded. Total scores range from 6 to 24, with higher scores reflecting more positive feelings of self-worth. The total score on the GSW is divided by six (the number of items comprising the subscale), thus resulting in a subscale mean item score ranging from 1 to 4. Normative and psychometric data for this scale are available for children in grades three through eight. Acceptable internal consistency coefficients for the GSW ranging from .78 to .84 have been reported by Harter (1985).

Lastly, the Child Coping Efficacy Scale (CCES; New Beginnings Codebook, 1992) is a 7-item scale designed to determine children's self-perceived efficacy of coping. This scale includes items regarding the extent to which children think their coping has been successful and how well they will be able to handle problems as they arise in the future. Three items that were present-oriented were included in analyses for this study. The coefficient alpha for this scale for a sample of children of divorce (ages 9-13) was .74.

In this study we reasoned that the ability to predict various coping styles would not only inform future intervention efforts but would also identify those factors most likely to predict adaptive and maladaptive coping efforts. With reference to avoidance coping, we hypothesized that it would be positively related to the amount of loss, and impact of negative life events, and negatively related to coping efficacy, perceived level of social support, and self-worth. The selection of these hypothesized predictors was based upon the notion that ways of coping are highly dependent upon availability of resources (Lazarus & Folkman, 1984) as well as the idea that recovery is dependent upon an individual's ability to reverse losses through the successful employment of remaining internal and external resources (Freedy, Saladin, Kilpatrick, & Resnick 1994; Hobfoll, 1991).

Results showed that within this sample of 92 youth there were no significant differences in the use or frequency of coping strategies. Two sets of hierarchical regression analyses were conducted to address how the same set of variables predicted the two types of coping strategies (avoidant and distraction). The predictors were entered in the following order: total resource loss, demographic variables (sex, age, race, and age × race interaction), impact of negative life events, social support, self-worth, and coping efficacy. Although situational variables, particularly coping efficacy, provided greater prediction of coping than did dispositional variables, both distraction and avoidance coping strategies were positively related to loss and impact of negative life events (see Tables 3 and 4). It should be noted however, that these relationships were not significant when controlling for other variables. In that few differences were found for the predictors of coping, we are presently examining the direct effects of only resource loss, coping efficacy, and social support on coping. Additionally, both mediational and moderational models that may explicate the relationship between resource loss and coping are being pursued.

Additionally, given that youths' reports were obtained approximately three months following the fire, consistent with the assertion made by Cummings and Cummings (1988), we determined it essential to examine the after-effects of exposure over extended periods of time (6, 12 and 24 months). In doing so, we hope to identify the interactive role of exposure and coping. Hence, a major conclusion from this study is the need to examine predictors of coping as direct effects as well as mediators and moderators. Examination of such predictors should also be car-

TABLE 3. Hierarchical Regression for Variance in Avoidance Coping

| | | Set statistics | | | Decomposition of set effect | | |
|---|---|---|---|---|---|---|---|
| Step | Variables | $R^2$ change | $R^2$ total | p | Beta | Unique $R^2$ | p |
| 1 | Loss | .08 | .08 | .00 | .29 | .08 | .00 |
| 2 | Demographic | .05 | .14 | .24 | | | |
| | Sex | | | | −.08 | .00 | .41 |
| | Race | | | | −.39 | .00 | .34 |
| | Age | | | | −.24 | .02 | .11 |
| | Race × Age | | | | .61 | .01 | .17 |
| 3 | Negative Life Events | .00 | .14 | .81 | .02 | .00 | .81 |
| 4 | Social Support | .00 | .14 | .76 | .03 | .00 | .766 |
| 5 | Self Worth | .01 | .16 | .24 | −.12 | .01 | .24 |
| 6 | Coping Efficacy | .07 | .23 | .00 | .31 | .07 | .00 |

TABLE 4. Hierarchical Regression for Variance in Distraction Strategies

| | | Set statistics | | | Decomposition of set effect | | |
|---|---|---|---|---|---|---|---|
| Step | Variables | $R^2$ change | $R^2$ total | p | Beta | Unique $R^2$ | p |
| 1 | Loss | .06 | .06 | .01 | .25 | .06 | .01 |
| 2 | Demographic | .05 | .11 | .27 | | | |
| | Sex | | | | .19 | .03 | .06 |
| | Race | | | | .25 | .00 | .55 |
| | Age | | | | −.00 | <.00 | .98 |
| | Race × Age | | | | −.25 | .00 | .57 |
| 3 | Negative Life Events | .02 | .14 | .13 | .16 | .02 | .13 |
| 4 | Social Support | .01 | .16 | .17 | .14 | .01 | .17 |
| 5 | Self Worth | .00 | .16 | .78 | .03 | .00 | .78 |
| 6 | Coping Efficacy | .04 | .20 | .02 | .24 | .04 | .02 |

ried out longitudinally. We are currently exploring these issues in our longitudinal data set.

# CONCLUSION

In summary, the conceptualization and systematic examination of risk factors in children and adolescents in the disaster area remains in its infancy. From a basic science perspective, understanding and appreciating the separate and interactive roles of these factors is essential if meaningful linkages between disasters and psychological adjustment are to be established. It is hoped that further study of avoidance coping and other risk factors, as well as coping efficacy and other protective factors, will assist investigators in developing intervention strategies that will result in better coping among children and adolescents in disaster situations.

Recommendations based on work with residential fires include the following:

1. The placement of risk factors into meaningful, conceptual categories may be helpful. For example, the contexts provided by Wenar and Kerig (2000), including organic, intrapersonal, interpersonal, and superordinate appear to be of heuristic importance.

2. The placement of risk factors into the appropriate temporal sequence in the context of disaster might also prove useful. That is, no systematic effort has been undertaken to more precisely place each of these groups of factors in the three phases of a disaster event: before, during, or after. Nor has anyone specified the degree to which each may cut across all three phases of the disaster experience.

3. Attention to terminological inconsistencies may lead to further progress in the disaster area. For example, greater clarity regarding the terms "risk factor" and "vulnerability factor" is called for, given that few investigators have precisely differentiated the two. As aptly pointed out by Wenar and Kerig (2000) "while risk may determine disturbance directly, vulnerability is the term used for factors that intensify the response to risk" (p. 20). In the context of disaster, for example, a risk factor may be defined as elevated levels of exposure to fire, while a vulnerability factor might be identified as gender or age of the child. That is, while both boys and girls are at risk for distress following exposure to fire, girls often report higher levels of distress (Jones & Ollendick, 2002). So too do younger children in comparison to older children. While the exact mechanisms associated with these findings are not fully understood at this time, this differentiation is important in that it may enable investigators to provide a finer level of analysis of the "dose-response" relationship as well as the relative roles of mediating and moderating variables. That is, for example, rather than studying gender as a risk factor, sex of the child should more ap-

propriately be viewed as a vulnerability factor where its interactional nature is then examined.
4. The need to better identify intervention efforts aimed at assisting
those impacted by disaster is apparent. A major goal of our work
has been the development of interventions to assist victimized
children, adolescents, and their parents to cope with the consequences of fire-related trauma. We have developed and evaluated
a number of behavioral and cognitive behavioral interventions for
children and their families targeting prevention at the primary,
secondary, and tertiary levels. Strategies have ranged from teaching fire evacuation skills (Jones, Kazdin & Haney, 1981) to mod-
eling anxiety reduction employing "Rehearsal-Plus" (Jones &
Randall, 1994). Inadvertently, these strategies have been aimed at
reducing avoidance behaviors and enhancing self-efficacy of these
children. However, the link between these variables and treatment
outcome are yet to be fully examined.

## REFERENCES

Ayers, T.S. Sandler, I.N., West, S.G., & Roosa, M.W. (1996). A dispositional and situational assessment of children's coping: Testing alternative models of coping. *Journal of Personality, 64*, 923-958.
Bandura, A. (1986). *Social foundations of thought and action.* New Jersey: Prentice
Hall.
Bandura, A. (1997). *Self-efficacy: The exercise of control.* New York: W. H. Freeman.
Benight, C., Ironson, G., Klebe, K., Carver, C.S., Wynings, C., Burnett, K., Green-
wood, D., Baum, A., & Schneiderman, N. (1998). Conservation of resources and
coping self-efficacy predicting distress following a natural disaster: A causal model
analysis where the environment meets the mind. *Journal of Anxiety, Stress, & Cop-
ing, 12*, 107-112.
Brand, A.H., & Johnson, J.H. (1982). Note on reliability of the Life Events Checklist.
*Psychological Reports, 50*, 1274.
Cummings, E.M., & Cummings, J.L. (1988). A process-oriented approach to children's coping with adults' angry behavior. *Developmental Review, 8*, 296-321.
Davies, P.T., & Cummings, E.M. (1995). Children's emotions as organizers of their reactions to interadult anger: A functionalist perspective. *Developmental Psychology,
31*, 677-684.
Dubow, E.F., & Ullman, D.G. (1989). Assessing social support in elementary school
children: The Survey of Children's Social Support. *Journal of Clinical Child Psychology, 18*, 52-64.
Freedy, J.R., Shaw, D.L., Jarrell, M.P., & Masters, C.R. (1992). Towards an understanding of the psychological impact of natural disasters: An application of the Conservation of Resource model. *Journal of Traumatic Stress, 5*, 441-454.

Freedy, J.R, Saladin, M.E, Kilpatrick, D.G, & Resnick, H.S. (1994). Understanding acute psychological distress following natural disaster. *Journal of Traumatic Stress, 7,* 257-273.

Harter, S. (1985). The Self-Perception Profile for Children: Revision of the Perceived Competence Scale for Children. Denver, CO: University of Denver.

Hobfoll, S.E. (1991). Traumatic stress: A theory based on rapid loss of resources. *Anxiety Research, 4,* 187-197.

Hollingshead, A.B. (1975). *Four Factor Index of Social Status.* New Haven, CT: privately printed.

Holmbeck, G. (1997). Toward terminological, conceptual, and statistical clarity in the study of mediators and moderators: Examples from the child-clinical and pediatric psychology literatures. *Journal of Consulting and Clinical Psychology, 65,* 599-614.

Johnson, J.H., & McCutcheon, S.M. (1980). Assessing life stress in older children and adolescents: Preliminary findings with the Life Events Checklist. In I.G. Sarason & C.D. Spielberger (Eds.), *Stress and anxiety* (Vol. 7, pp. 111-125). Washington, DC: Hemisphere.

Jones, R.T., & Ollendick, T.H. (2002). The impact of residential fire on children and their families. In A. La Greca, W. Sliverman, E. Vernberg, & M. Roberts (Eds.), *Helping children cope with disasters: Integrating research and practice* (pp. 175-202). Washington, DC: American Psychological Association Books.

Jones, R.T., Wang, Y., & Ollendick, T.H. (in preparation). Predictors of coping strategies following residential fire. Virginia Polytechnic Institute and State University.

Jones, R.T., Kazdin, A.E., & Haney, J. (1981). Social validation and training of emergency fire safety skills for potential injury prevention and life saving. *Journal of Applied Behavior Analysis, 14,* 249-260.

Jones, R.T., & Randall, J. (1994). Rehearsal-Plus: Coping with fire emergencies and reducing fire-related fears. *Fire Technology, 30,* 432-444.

Kaslow, N.J., Tanenbaum, R.L., & Seligman, M.E.P. (1978). The KASTAN-R: A children's attributional style questionnaire (KASTAN-R-CASQ). Unpublished manuscript.

Kliewer, W., & Lewis, H. (1995). Family influences on coping processes in children and adolescents with sickle cell disease. *Journal of Pediatric Psychology, 20,* 511-525.

Lazarus, R.S., & Folkman, S. (1984). *Stress, appraisal and coping.* New York: Springer.

McKernon, W.L., Holmbeck, G.N., Colder, C.R., Hommeyer, J.S., Shapera, W., & Westhoven, V. (2001). Longitudinal study of observed and perceived family influences on problem-focused coping behaviors of preadolescents with spina bifida. *Journal of Pediatric Psychology, 26,* 41-54.

New Beginnings Codebook (1992). Unpublished manuscript. Tempe, AZ: Arizona State University.

Ollendick, T.H. (1983). Reliability and validity of the Revised Fear Survey Schedule for Children (FSSC-R). *Behaviour Research and Therapy, 21,* 685-692.

Ollendick, T.H., Langley, A.K., Jones, R.T., & Kephart, C. (2001). Fear in children and adolescents: Relations with negative life events, attributional style, and avoidant coping. *Journal of Child Psychological Psychiatry, 42,* 1029-1034.

Pfefferbaum, B. (1997). Posttraumatic stress disorder in children: A review of the past 10 years. *Journal of the American Academy of Child and Adolescent Psychiatry, 36,* 1503-1511.

Saigh, P.A., & Bremner, J.D. (1999). *Posttraumatic stress disorder: A comprehensive text.* Boston: Allyn & Bacon.

Sandler, I.N., Tein, J., & West, S.C. (1994). Coping, stress, and the psychological symptoms of children of divorce: A cross-sectional and longitudinal study. *Child Development, 65,* 1744-1763.

Skinner, E.A., Edge, K., Altman, J., & Sheerwood, H. (2003). Searching for the structure of coping: A review and critique of category systems for classifying ways of coping. *Psychological Bulletin, 129*(2), 216-269.

Steele, R.G., Forehand, R., & Armistead, L. (1997). The role of family processes and coping strategies in the relationship between parental chronic illness and childhood internalizing problems. *Journal of Abnormal Child Psychology, 25,* 83-94.

Thompson, R.J., Kronenberger, W.G., Johnson, D.R., & Whiting, K. (1989). The role of central nervous system functioning and family functioning in behavioral problems of children with myelodysplasia, *Developmental and Behavioral Pediatrics 10,* 242-248.

Wenar, C., & Kerig, P. (2000). *Developmental psychopathology: From infancy through adolescence.* Boston: McGraw-Hill.

# Treatment of Acute Traumatic Stress Reactions

## David Spiegel, MD

**SUMMARY.** This paper calls for a broadening of the context within which we study responses to traumatic stress, the course of recovery, components of effective interventions, and assessments of outcome. Acute stress reactions to trauma as a spectrum include anxiety, dissociative, and depressive symptoms. The course of these symptoms may vary, with fluctuations between intrusion ("positive") and avoidance/numbing/dissociative ("negative") symptoms that may complicate assessment, treatment-seeking, and course of recovery. Components of effective treatments including affect management, cognitive restructuring, and social integration are discussed. Finally, a broader view of outcome assessment in such research is called for, including not just reduction in psychopathological symptoms but attention to coping styles, affect management, resilience, social reorganization, and sensitivity to subsequent trauma. *[Article copies available for a fee from The Haworth Document Delivery Service: 1-800-HAWORTH. E-mail address: <docdelivery@haworthpress.com> Website: <http://www.HaworthPress.com> © 2005 by The Haworth Press, Inc. All rights reserved.]*

**KEYWORDS.** Acute stress, ASD, treatment, intervention

David Spiegel is Professor of Psychiatry & Behavioral Sciences, Stanford University, Stanford, CA.

Address correspondence to: David Spiegel, MD, Professor of Psychiatry & Behavioral Sciences, Stanford University School of Medicine, 401 Quarry Road, Stanford, CA 94305-5718 (E-mail: dspiegel@leland.stanford.edu).

[Haworth co-indexing entry note]: "Treatment of Acute Traumatic Stress Reactions." Spiegel, David. Co-published simultaneously in *Journal of Trauma & Dissociation* (The Haworth Medical Press, an imprint of The Haworth Press, Inc.) Vol. 6, No. 2, 2005, pp. 101-108; and: *Acute Reactions to Trauma and Psychotherapy: A Multidisciplinary and International Perspective* (ed: Etzel Cardeña, and Kristin Croyle) The Haworth Medical Press, an imprint of The Haworth Press, Inc., 2005, pp. 101-108. Single or multiple copies of this article are available for a fee from The Haworth Document Delivery Service [1-800-HAWORTH, 9:00 a.m. - 5:00 p.m. (EST). E-mail address: docdelivery@haworthpress.com].

Available online at http://www.haworthpress.com/web/JTD
© 2005 by The Haworth Press, Inc. All rights reserved.
doi:10.1300/J229v06n02_09

Acute stress disorder (ASD) represents a challenge to those with the disorder, to mental health professionals, and to those involved in public policy. The substantial minority of individuals who suffer these symptoms may recover spontaneously, but a considerable proportion will go on to develop post-traumatic stress disorder (PTSD), and could potentially benefit substantially from expert help. Research on the treatment of ASD constitutes a laboratory for population-based as well as individual and group interventions.

The spectrum of symptomatology in ASD includes anxiety-based symptoms such as intrusive thoughts, nightmares, irritability, and restlessness; dissociative symptoms including numbness, amnesia, reliving, depersonalization, and derealization; and depressive symptoms, including a sense of foreshortened future and loss of pleasure. ASD was introduced as a category in *DSM-IV* to acknowledge the severity of symptomatology that may occur in the immediate aftermath of trauma. It is also predictive of PTSD in a number of studies (Brewin, Andrews, Rose, & Kirk, 1999; Cardeña, Koopman, Classen, & Spiegel, 1996; Classen, Koopman, Hales, & Spiegel, 1998; Koopman, Gore-Felton, & Spiegel, 1997; Staab, Grieger, Fullerton, & Ursano, 1996; Koopman, Classen, & Spiegel, 1994; Cardeña & Spiegel, 1993). While the incremental predictive power of ASD symptoms has been questioned (Bryant & Harvey, 1996; Harvey & Bryant, 1998; Marshall, Spitzer, & Liebowitz, 1999), several issues should be borne in mind. The predictive power of ASD for PTSD provided initial construct validity for ASD as a diagnosis, but is not the main reason for its existence. The fact that it predicts PTSD as well as it does, given the difference in symptom clusters, is in itself interesting. It may well be that dissociative symptoms occur more frequently in the immediate peritraumatic period, providing an initial adaptive response to acute stress (Butler, Duran, Jasiukatis, Koopman, & Spiegel, 1996; Foa & Hearst-Ikeda, 1996), that may become maladaptive over time by delaying necessary cognitive processing of traumatic events (Lindemann, 1994). Indeed, MacFarlane has shown that dissociative symptoms on the day of a motor vehicle accident do not predict PTSD 6 months later, but dissociation two weeks after the accident does (McFarlane, 1997).

Another consideration is that the current symptom cluster in PTSD is a less than ideal "gold standard" for post-traumatic symptomatology. In regard to dissociation, it contains numbing, avoidance, and reliving (dissociating the memory from current circumstances or the outcome of the traumatic experience). It may well under-represent the importance of dissociative symptoms. Indeed, the so-called "negative" symptoms of PTSD may be more problematic even if they often co-occur with intrusion and hyperarousal symptoms because they are less likely to call attention to themselves and thereby invite referral or treatment. Individuals who are avoidant, numb, amnesic, or lose pleasure in usually pleasurable activities may not realize the need for or seek help. Indeed they may not appear distressed, especially in comparison with those who manifest more nightmares, flashbacks, ruminative or hyperarousal symptoms after trauma. Numbing has long been found to be a strong predictor of the development of later PTSD, for example, among Israeli combat soliders (Solomon, Mikulincer, & Benbenishty, 1989) and in recent analysis of the Oklahoma City bombing data (North, 1999, 2001). Arieh Shalev found that peritraumatic dissociation predicted the development of PTSD (Shalev, Peri, Canetti, & Schreiber, 1996), although in more recent work he finds that depressive symptoms overcome the shared variance of dissociation in predicting PTSD outcome. Similar results are now being obtained among children, who are more prone to dissociation than adults (Lippmann & Steer, 1996).

## COURSE OF SYMPTOM RECOVERY

The ability of pre-diagnosis symptoms to predict PTSD symptoms is limited to at best about a third of the variance. Pre-trauma diagnosis also accounts for additional variance, as do at least two post-treatment variables: poor social support and subsequent stressors (Brewin et al., 1999). This provides a major opportunity for therapeutic interventions to potentially reduce PTSD symptoms by enhancing social support, providing substitute support, and by reducing exposure to subsequent stressors. There is evidence that dissociation in the immediate aftermath of trauma is associated with a tendency to endanger oneself, e.g., by crossing police barricades or engaging in irrelevant activities that do not promote safety during a crisis (Koopman, Classen, & Spiegel, 1996; Koopman, Classen, Spiegel, & Cardeña, 1995). Thus intervention could reduce risk behavior among those prone to it, and therefore subsequent retraumatization.

## COMPONENTS OF EFFECTIVE INTERVENTIONS

Any intervention that has the power to help has the power to hurt. There has been considerable controversy about the efficacy of critical incident stress debriefing (Kenardy et al., 1996; Wollman, 1993). A Cochrane database review indicated no specific efficacy for it, and a recent review by Foa and colleagues (Foa & Meadows, 1997; Wollman, 1993) found that in some circumstances CISD might actually worsen outcome, especially among those with high initial symptom levels. Two components of many stress-debriefing approaches that have the potential to be toxic are:

1. The anticipation of future emotional problems. In the immediate aftermath of trauma, the last thing trauma victims want or need to hear is the prediction of future difficulties. The present ones are quite enough. Indeed such predictions may induce rather than prevent certain emotional reactions.
2. Many of these interventions are quite brief–lasting perhaps an hour to ninety minutes, and occurring only once. They may have the effect of stirring up emotional reactions without providing any means for restructuring the meaning of the emotional experiences and traumatic events, enhancing skill at regulating emotional response, or providing a supportive social environment for managing the emotion.

Future research on the therapeutic elements of treating acute trauma would benefit from a broad conceptual framework. Rather than simply building on the theoretical traditions from which investigators came, e.g., cognitive-behavioral, psychodynamic, educational, existential, it would help to identify common therapeutic elements in diverse therapies that have either positive, little, or adverse effects on outcome. If the essence of trauma is helplessness, therapeutic interventions can be understood from the perspective of their ability to enhance control over specific symptoms or problems. Candidate dimensions are the following:

1. *Emotion.* Emotional intelligence, emotional expression, emotional self-efficacy, and emotional disposition are all-important facets of trauma response and components of effective interventions. Traumatic memories come associated with strong emotion, and means of ventilating, coming to terms with, and managing strong emotion are critical to good psychotherapeutic support (Lindemann, 1994).
2. *Cognitive restructuring.* Many effective therapies help traumatized individuals to examine their memories and experiences from

a new point of view, allowing them to find new meaning in the experience. They may, for example, come to recognize their good fortune in surviving the trauma, to acknowledge something they did to protect themselves or others, or to realize that they were not responsible for the traumatic event that befell them (Spiegel, 1996; Spiegel, 1997; Spiegel & Classen, 1996). Effective techniques for doing this range from videotapes for rape victims prior to their medical examination to cognitive therapies (Foa & Meadows, 1997; Resick, Jordan, Girelli, Hutter, & Marhoefer-Dvorak, 1988). Effective techniques in this domain range from simple information provision to profound cognitive restructuring.

3. *Symptom management.* Many interventions involve teaching how to control symptoms of hyperarousal and somatic distress that accompanies intrusive recollections of trauma or exposure to reminders of traumatic experiences, including imaginal desensitization (Foa & Meadows, 1997) and hypnosis (Spiegel, 1995, 1996).

4. *Social support.* Studies of the social context of trauma treatment are crucial. Examination of effects of individual versus group intervention, treatment involving families, schools, co-workers, communities and other natural social groupings are critical. Western societies tend to be heavily focused on the individual, while Eastern cultures are much more sociocentric. The nature of interventions in their social context requires considerable research. While some interventions may only be effective in a given cultural context, there may be lessons to be learned from diverse cultures, especially in the social dimension of therapeutic support. The study of treatment relationships should include traumatic transference issues involved in the therapy (Spiegel, 1996), and how therapeutic interaction can be used to model impact of trauma on outside relationships and the potential to improve them.

5. *Timing.* The timing of intervention in relation to the traumatic experience requires further research.

6. *Dose.* The extent of treatment sessions and how many of them are provided are important dimensions of therapeutic structure that requires research.

7. *Individual characteristics.* The characteristics that predispose a person to good or poor therapeutic outcome should be studied.

8. *Therapist characteristics.* The characteristics of therapists that are associated with good outcome, such as training and experience, should be examined.

## OUTCOME

Outcome variables assessing treatment response should be broadened. While reduction of PTSD symptoms is important, it should not be the only outcome dimension studied. Other salient domains include other psychiatric symptoms such as depressive and dissociative symptoms and substance abuse. Other domains of coping and resiliency should also be studied, such as emotional self-efficacy, emotional expression, and decreased emotional control (Giese-Davis et al., 2002) and anger management.

Dimensions often overlooked in evaluating treatment outcome include relationship management, especially given the often profound effects of ASD and PTSD on existing and new relationships. A related outcome variable is interrupting the all too common cycle of sexual and physical abuse. In addition, since trauma and post-traumatic symptoms seem to sensitize individuals to trauma, effects of intervention on subsequent traumatic stress management should be studied.

## CONCLUSION

A large and growing number of disciplines are involved in acute trauma treatment research. We should draw on this expanding group of investigators to enlarge the nomological net of trauma treatment research. Rather than limit or defend domains of interest, we should expand them in a search for a more complete understanding of the domain of acute trauma-induced problems and means of helping people cope with them. Let us in the trauma research field avoid "hierarchical regression" and expand multivariate investigation of acute trauma treatment process and outcome.

## REFERENCES

Brewin, C.R., Andrews, B., Rose, S., & Kirk, M. (1999). Acute stress disorder and posttraumatic stress disorder in victims of violent crime [see comments]. *American Journal of Psychiatry*, *156*(3), 360-366.

Bryant, R.A., & Harvey, A.G. (1996). Initial posttraumatic stress responses following motor vehicle accidents. *Journal of Traumatic Stress*, *9*, 223-234.

Butler, L.D., Duran, E.F.D., Jasiukatis, P., Koopman, C., & Spiegel, D. (1996). Hypnotizability and traumatic experience: A diathesis-stress model of dissociative symptomatology. *American Journal of Psychiatry*, *153*, 42-63.

Cardeña, E., Koopman, C., Classen, C., & Spiegel, D. (1996). Psychometric review of the Stanford Acute Stress Reaction Questionnaire (SASRQ). In B. Stamm (Ed.), *Measurement of stress, trauma, and adaptation* (pp. 293-297). Lutherville: Sidran Press.

Cardeña, E., & Spiegel, D. (1993). Dissociative reactions to the San Francisco Bay Area earthquake of 1989. *American Journal of Psychiatry, 150,* 474-478.

Classen, C., Koopman, C., Hales, R., & Spiegel, D. (1998). Acute stress disorder as a predictor of posttraumatic stress symptoms. *American Journal of Psychiatry, 155,* 620-624.

Foa, E.B., & Hearst-Ikeda, D. (1996). Emotional dissociation in response to trauma. In L.K. Michelson & W.J. Ray (Eds.), *Handbook of dissociation* (pp. 207-226). New York: Plenum.

Foa, E.B., & Meadows, E.A. (1997). Psychosocial treatments for posttraumatic stress disorder: A critical review. *Annual Review of Psychology, 48,* 449-480.

Giese-Davis, J., Koopman, C., Butler, L., Classen, C., Cordova, M., Fobair, P., Benson, J., Kraemer, H., & Spiegel, D. (2002). Change in emotion-regulation strategy for women with metastatic breast cancer following supportive-expressive group therapy. *Journal of Consulting and Clinical Psychology, 70,* 916-925.

Harvey, A.G., & Bryant, R.A. (1998). Relationship between acute stress disorder and posttraumatic stress disorder: A prospective evaluation of motor vehicle accident survivors. *Journal of Consulting and Clinical Psychology, 66,* 507-512.

Kenardy, J.A., Webster, R.A., Lewin, T.J., Carr, V.J., Hazell, P.L., & Carter, G.L. (1996). Stress debriefing and patterns of recovery following a natural disaster. *Journal of Traumatic Stress, 9,* 37-49.

Koopman, C., Classen, C., & Spiegel, D. (1994). Predictors of posttraumatic stress symptoms among survivors of the Oakland/Berkeley, Calif., firestorm. *American Journal of Psychiatry, 151,* 888-894.

Koopman, C., Classen, C., & Spiegel, D. (1996). Dissociative responses in the immediate aftermath of the Oakland/Berkeley Firestorm. *Journal of Traumatic Stress, 9,* 521-540.

Koopman, C., Classen, C., Spiegel, D., & Cardeña, E. (1995). When disaster strikes, acute stress disorders may follow. *Journal of Traumatic Stress, 8,* 29-46.

Koopman, C., Gore-Felton, C., & Spiegel, D. (1997). Acute stress disorder symptoms among female sexual abuse survivors seeking treatment. *Journal of Child Sexual Abuse, 6*(3), 65-85.

Lindemann, E. (1994). Symptomatology and management of acute grief. *American Journal of Psychiatry, 151*(6 Supplement), 155-160.

Lippmann, J., & Steer, R. (1996). Sexually abused children suffering posttraumatic stress symptoms: Initial treatment outcome findings. *Child Maltreatment, 1,* 310-321.

Marshall, R.D., Spitzer, R., & Liebowitz, M.R. (1999). Review and critique of the new DSM-IV diagnosis of Acute Stress Disorder. *American Journal of Psychiatry, 156,* 1677-1685.

McFarlane, A. (1997). The prevalence and longitudinal course of PTSD: Implications for the neurobiological models of PTSD. In A.C. MacFarlane & R. Yehuda (Eds.),

*Psychobiology of posttraumatic stress disorder* (Annals of the New York Academy of Sciences, Vol. 821, pp. 10-23). New York: New York Academy of Science.

North, C.S. (1999). Psychiatric disorders among survivors of the Oklahoma City bombing. *JAMA, 282,* 755-762.

North, C.S. (2001). The course of post-traumatic stress disorder after the Oklahoma City bombing. *Military Medicine, 166*(12 Supplement), 51-52.

Resick, P.A., Jordan, C.G., Girelli, S.A., Hutter, C.K., & Marhoefer-Dvorak, S. (1988). A comparative outcome study of behavioral group therapy for sexual assault victims. *Behavior Therapy, 19,* 385-401.

Shalev, A.Y., Peri, T., Canetti, L., & Schreiber, S. (1996). Predictors of PTSD in injured trauma survivors: A prospective study. *American Journal of Psychiatry, 153,* 219-225.

Solomon, Z., Mikulincer, M., & Benbenishty, R. (1989). Combat stress reaction: Clinical manifestations and correlates. *Military Psychology, 1,* 35-47.

Spiegel, D. (1995). Hypnosis, dissociation, and trauma: Hidden and overt observers in repression and dissociation. In J.L. Singer (Ed.), *Repression and dissociation: Implications for personality theory, psychopathology, and health* (pp. 121-142). Chicago: University of Chicago Press.

Spiegel, D. (1996). Hypnosis in the treatment of Posttraumatic Stress Disorder. In S. Lynn & I. Kirsch & J. Rhue (Eds.), *Casebook of clinical hypnosis* (pp. 999-111). Washington DC: American Psychological Press.

Spiegel, D. (1997). Trauma, dissociation, and memory. *Annals of the New York Academy of Sciences, 821,* 225-237.

Spiegel, D., & Classen, C. (1996). Acute stress disorder. In G. Gabbard & S. Atkinson (Eds.), *Synopsis of treatments of psychiatric disorders* (2nd ed., pp. 655-666). Washington DC: American Psychiatric Press.

Staab, J.P., Grieger, T.A., Fullerton, C.S., & Ursano, R.J. (1996). Acute stress disorder, subsequent posttraumatic stress disorder and depression after a series of typhoons. *Anxiety, 2*(5), 219-225.

Wollman, D. (1993). Critical incident stress debriefing and crisis groups: A review of the literature. *GROUP, 17*(2), 70-83.

# Treating Traumatized Children:
# Current Status and Future Directions

Judith A. Cohen, MD

**SUMMARY.** Empirical knowledge regarding effective treatments for traumatized children has increased in the past decade, yet much still remains unknown. There is growing support for the efficacy of trauma-focused cognitive behavioral therapy (TF-CBT) for treating PTSD, depressive, and behavioral problems in sexually abused children, and evidence that suggests that this treatment is effective for children exposed to other types of trauma, and for multiply traumatized children. Few other psychosocial treatments have been adequately studied to date. Open psychopharmacological studies have identified several promising medication classes for traumatized children but these need to be tested in randomized, placebo controlled trials. No empirical studies have evaluated the efficacy of early interventions provided to children in the acute aftermath of mass disasters or terrorist acts. More research is needed to test potentially effective treatments for traumatized children, and to identify

Judith A. Cohen is Professor of Psychiatry, Drexel University College of Medicine, and Medical Director, Center for Traumatic Stress in Children and Adolescents, Allegheny General Hospital, Pittsburgh, PA.

Address correspondence to: Judith A. Cohen, MD, Allegheny General Hospital, Four Allegheny Center, 8th Floor, Pittsburgh, PA 15212 (E-mail: jcohen1@wpahs.org).

This paper was prepared in part with funding from grants from NIMH K02 MH01938 and SAMHSA SM54319.

The author gratefully acknowledges Anthony Mannarino, PhD, Lucy Berliner, MSW, and Ann Marie Kotlik for their contributions in the conceptualization and preparation of this paper.

[Haworth co-indexing entry note]: "Treating Traumatized Children: Current Status and Future Directions." Cohen, Judith A. Co-published simultaneously in *Journal of Trauma & Dissociation* (The Haworth Medical Press, an imprint of The Haworth Press, Inc.) Vol. 6, No. 2, 2005, pp. 109-121; and: *Acute Reactions to Trauma and Psychotherapy: A Multidisciplinary and International Perspective* (ed: Etzel Cardeña, and Kristin Croyle) The Haworth Medical Press, an imprint of The Haworth Press, Inc., 2005, pp. 109-121. Single or multiple copies of this article are available for a fee from The Haworth Document Delivery Service [1-800-HAWORTH, 9:00 a.m. - 5:00 p.m. (EST). E-mail address: docdelivery@haworthpress.com].

optimal methods for disseminating and implementing evidence-based treatments to community practitioners.*[Article copies available for a fee from The Haworth Document Delivery Service: 1-800-HAWORTH. E-mail address: <docdelivery@haworthpress.com> Website: <http://www.HaworthPress.com>*

KEYWORDS. Treatment, trauma, posttraumatic stress disorder, PTSD, children

Research in the past decade has produced an impressive growth in our knowledge about effective treatments for traumatized children and adolescents. As a result, we have successfully identified at least one effective psychosocial treatment approach (trauma-focused cognitive behavioral therapy; TF-CBT) for this population. Several open label medication treatment trials have also been published which offer the potential of additional effective early interventions for children exposed to traumatic life events. This paper will briefly review the progress that has been made in this regard, and discuss aspects of treating traumatized children, who have been poorly studied and require additional resources and research.

## CURRENT KNOWLEDGE ABOUT PSYCHOSOCIAL TREATMENTS

Several types of psychosocial interventions are currently provided to traumatized children in the U.S. According to one national survey of practitioners specializing in treating this population, non-physician treatment providers prefer cognitive behavioral, family and play therapies, while physician providers prefer pharmacologic, psychodynamic and cognitive behavioral therapies for the treatment of childhood posttraumatic stress disorder (PTSD; Cohen, Mannarino, & Rogal, 2001). Of these treatments, TF-CBT has garnered the most empirical support; six randomized clinical trials and several less rigorously controlled studies have demonstrated that TF-CBT is superior to play therapy, supportive therapy, standard community treatment, or wait list control conditions in decreasing PTSD and other trauma-related symptoms in children from 3-18 years of age (reviewed in Cohen, Berliner, & March,

2000; Cohen, Deblinger, Mannarino & Steer, 2004; Cohen, Mannarino & Knudsen, 2005; King et al., 2002).

Other forms of trauma-focused treatments have limited evidence of efficacy in treating traumatized children. Play therapy provided in either group or individual settings, was found in one randomized clinical trial, to be superior to a no-treatment control condition in improving self-concept and self-mastery in sexually abused children (Perez, 1988). Family therapy was found to be equally effective as CBT, with both of these treatments being superior to community treatment as usual in decreasing children's externalizing and violent behaviors, in one randomized clinical trial for physically abused children (Kolko, 1996). Another study for parents of physically abused children used a modified version of Parent-Child Interactional Therapy (PCIT) and found that PCIT was superior to a parenting group in decreasing physically abusive parenting behaviors (Chaffin et al., 2004). A specialized form of CBT, eye movement desensitization and reprocessing (EMDR), in which therapist-directed eye movements accompany standard CBT techniques, was found in one study to be superior to a wait list control condition for reducing PTSD symptoms in youths exposed to a hurricane (Chemtob, Nakashima & Carlson, 2002) and in another to be comparable to TF-CBT for sexually abused girls (Jaberghaderi, Greenwald, Rubin, Dolatabadim, & Zand, 2002). Massage therapy was also superior to a video control condition in reducing PTSD symptoms in children exposed to a hurricane (Field, Seligman, Scafedi, & Schanberg, 1996). Psychodynamic psychotherapy was found to be superior to psychoeducation therapy in another randomized clinical trial (Trowell et al., 2002); but, because psychodynamic treatment was provided individually for 30 sessions and the psychoeducation was provided in a group format for 15 sessions, it is not clear whether the type, format or dosage was responsible for differential treatment response. Although replication studies are needed to confirm these findings, they offer preliminary support for a variety of psychosocial treatments for traumatized children.

Numerous open treatment trials (i.e., those without random assignment and with no comparison or control condition) have also been published, but these types of trials provide less information about treatment efficacy, as it is impossible to ascertain whether improvements came from the specific treatment provided, from non-specific aspects of treatment, or simply the passage of time. Other treatments such as crisis intervention ("psychological debriefing," critical incident stress debriefing) have produced conflicting results in adults, with some studies showing a detrimental effect of such interventions (Bisson, McFarlane & Rose,

2000) but have not yet been empirically evaluated in children. As will be discussed below, this is also a concern for pharmacologic treatments.

## CURRENT KNOWLEDGE
## ABOUT PSYCHOPHARMACOLOGIC TREATMENTS

Despite the fact that many traumatized children are apparently receiving psychopharmacological interventions (Foa, Davidson, & Frances, 1999), there has only been one randomized trial evaluating the efficacy of any medication in this population. In this study, acutely burned children with Acute Stress Disorder were randomized to receive either the tricyclic antidepressant imipramine, or the sedative medication chloral hydrate (Robert, Blakeney, Villarreal, Rosenberg, & Meyer, 1999). The group receiving imipramine was significantly less likely to develop PTSD, suggesting that this medication may be helpful in preventing the development of this disorder in this population. Unfortunately tricyclic antidepressant medications are associated with rare but serious cardiac side effects, which limit their current usefulness. In addition, burn victims have significant physiological abnormalities which may limit the generalizability of these findings to other traumatized children.

Various medications have been tested in open treatment trials for traumatized children, including those that act on the adrenergic (propranolol, clonidine, guanfacine), dopaminergic (risperidol), opiate (morphine), and kindling (carbamazepine) systems of the brain. However, children have a particularly high rate of placebo response, and many psychotropic medications that appear to be effective when used in open treatment trials are subsequently found to be no better than placebo when subjected to double blind randomized clinical trials (RCT). Likewise, it is inadvisable to extrapolate findings from adult studies onto children and adolescents, as differences in brain development, drug metabolism, and other factors differentiate these populations (Birmaher, Ryan, Brent, Williamson, & Kaufman, 1996). Thus, until placebo controlled RCTs are available, it is premature to conclude that any pharmacologic treatments effectively treat PTSD and other trauma symptoms in children or adolescents.

## LIMITATIONS OF OUR CURRENT KNOWLEDGE

Despite recent advances in treatment research for traumatized children, there are many limitations to our current knowledge. These limitations include: inadequate studies of most types of psychotherapies including those provided in the acute aftermath of mass disasters; the lack of dismantling studies for the one treatment (TF-CBT) with demonstrated efficacy for this population; limited treatment studies for children traumatized by different types of events; the lack of rigorous psychopharmacologic and combined psychotherapy-psychopharmacologic treatment trials; and the lack of treatment research for children and adolescents with comorbid psychiatric conditions or chronic, "complex PTSD" symptoms.

## Limited Psychotherapy Studies

Of all of the current psychotherapeutic models used to treat traumatized children, only TF-CBT and community care as usual have received adequate empirical evaluation to evaluate efficacy (i.e., at least two replication RCT studies performed by independent research teams). Most other types of treatment have only been examined in one or two treatment trials by a single research team, or not at all. Typically these treatment trials have been quite small; in some cases the comparison treatments used were not adequately defined or differentiated from the index treatment, or the studies have been inadequately powered to detect differential treatment effects even if such effects were present. Both positive and negative results of such trials need to be replicated in order to know whether such trials were truly representative of the efficacy of the treatment being studied. It is important to design appropriate trials of a variety of treatment approaches. Otherwise, there is a risk of finding the greatest efficacy for the treatments most easily manualized and subjected to empirical evaluation, simply because they are easier to study.

Although there is growing evidence that TF-CBT models are efficacious in decreasing PTSD and other trauma-related symptoms in children and adolescents, there is little information on which specific components of this treatment model are most critical to recovery. It is not clear whether the same components are necessary for all children, or whether some children (based on developmental level, symptom severity or which PTSD symptom cluster predominates) respond just as well without receiving all TF-CBT components. For example, there may be a subgroup of traumatized children for whom creating a detailed trauma narrative ("gradual exposure") is unnecessary, or even deleterious. Dismantling studies that examine the different components of CBT are needed to address these questions. Additionally, there is no information about optimal treatment dosage, that is, how many treatment sessions over what period of time is optimal for symptom remission or return to normal functioning. In this regard, most treatment studies consider remission from full syndromal disorder to be evidence of treatment efficacy. Few studies have included adequate measures of adaptive functioning, i.e., what proportion of children recover to the point of normal functioning. Since the latter is the presumed optimal goal of treatment, more attention to this aspect of treatment response is warranted.

## Limited Treatment Studies for Different Types of Traumatic Events

The majority of treatment studies for traumatized children have utilized sexually abused cohorts. While many of these children have experienced more chronic, intentional and personalized trauma than other traumatized children (and thus may represent highly symptomatic and/or difficult to treat cohorts), it is not clear that effective treatments for this group would necessarily be optimal for children exposed to other types of trauma. For example, it may be that the issues of stigmatization and shame, which are so relevant and predictive of psychopathology in sexually abused children, may be less critical to children traumatized by motor vehicle accidents or cancer. The psychological impact on non-offending parents of one's child being sexually abused suggests that inclusion of parents in treatment for this population is crucial; the empirical evidence for these children supports this approach (Cohen & Mannarino, 2000; Deblinger, Lippman, & Steer, 1996). It is expected that children experiencing other types of trauma which impact greatly on family members, such as domestic violence or traumatic death of a parent or sibling, will similarly require the inclusion of parents in treatment for optimal treatment response. A recently completed randomized controlled trial with 229 abused children suggested that these groups overlap to a significant extent. Although sexual abuse was the presenting trauma for these children, 70% of this cohort had been confronted with traumatic news such as the sudden death of a family member, 58% had experienced domestic violence and 26% had been physically abused (Cohen et al., 2004). In addition to these ongoing or interpersonal traumas, 37% had witnessed or been involved in a serious accident, 17% were witnesses or victims of community violence, 14% had experienced a fire or natural disaster, and 25% had experienced other PTSD-type traumas. These children experienced a mean of 3.6 different *types* of traumatic life events. The finding that TF-CBT was superior to supportive child centered therapy for these children suggests that this treatment is likely to be effective for a variety of childhood traumas, as well as for multiply traumatized children.

Most studies for children exposed to ongoing interpersonal violence such as sexual abuse, physical abuse or domestic violence, have included active parental treatment components. However, children exposed to community violence have responded well to school-based CBT interventions in two randomized trials which did not include a parental treatment component (Stein et al., 2003; Kataoka et al., 2003). Similarly, children experiencing single episode traumas, or adolescents exposed to war conditions have in open treatment trials appeared to respond well to group CBT interventions without parental treatment (Layne et al., 2001; March, Amaya-Jackson, Murray, & Schulte, 1998). Two randomized treatment trials for children exposed to natural disasters similarly did not require parental involvement to produce differential treatment outcomes (Chemtob, Nakashima & Hamada, 2002; Field et al., 1996). Randomized clinical trials for children exposed to a variety of traumatic stressors are needed. In addition, studies that evaluate the efficacy of early treatments (for example, those typically provided in the immediate aftermath of mass disasters) are also needed.

## Lack of Controlled Pharmacologic and Combined Psychotherapy-Pharmacologic Studies

As noted above, there are serious limitations inherent in pharmacologic studies that do not include random assignment and placebo control conditions. The expectation that taking medication will lead to a positive outcome is quite marked in children and parents, and this appears to be particularly true for children with psychiatric disorders. Similarly, studies that exclude the most symptomatic children, those with comorbid psychiatric conditions, or those who are not optimally compliant with treatment, are likely biased toward finding positive treatment results; additionally, they are not representative of children typically treated in routine clinical practice, so results from such studies may not be widely applicable. It is also essential to determine whether the addition of pharmacotherapy to psychosocial treatments such as TF-CBT will result in more timely, more complete, or longer lasting symptom remission, as medication and psychosocial treatments are often provided concurrently (Foa et al., 1999).

Trauma exposure and PTSD are typically under-recognized in primary care settings; early identification in routine care settings is critical, especially in light of the serious and potentially life-long changes in brain development recently documented in children exposed to abuse or domestic violence (DeBellis et al., 1999). It has been estimated that less than 2% of abused children with significant psychiatric symptoms receive any specialized treatment (Trupin, Tarico, & Low, 1993); this suggests that many traumatized children will be treated by primary care providers or not at all. The majority of this treatment will consist of pharmacotherapy, which is the predominant type of treatment provided by primary care providers for psychiatric conditions. Furthermore, among physicians specializing in treating traumatized children, almost 15% identified pharmacotherapy alone (i.e., not provided in conjunction with psychotherapy) as the first line treatment of choice for this population (Cohen et al., 2001). Given these trends, placebo controlled randomized trials are needed to determine whether such widespread prescribing practices are warranted for traumatized children.

## Lack of Treatment Studies for Children with Comorbid Psychiatric Conditions

Childhood PTSD is highly comorbid with other serious psychiatric disorders, including depression, other anxiety disorders, attention deficit-hyperactivity disorder (ADHD), conduct disorder and substance use disorders.There is growing evidence that left untreated, the presence of PTSD predisposes youth to developing depression, suicidality, substance use disorders and conduct disorders in youth and early adulthood (Silverman, Reinherz, & Giaconia, 1996; Warshaw et al., 1995). Yet all of the heretofore published treatment studies for childhood PTSD have excluded children with some or any of these comorbid disorders. In typical practice, such children may not receive services from trauma treatment programs because the severity of their other symptoms leads to the belief that they will not be able to benefit from such treatment until the comorbid condition is treated (Cohen, Mannarino, Zhitova, & Capone, 2003). Since such children have not typically been included in treatment trials, there are no data to support or challenge this practice.

Similarly, the term "complex PTSD" has been used to refer to children and adolescents exposed to chronic overwhelming trauma, and who have serious functional impairments in multiple domains (social, academic, cognitive, affective, self-injury, medical, etc.). Children and youth with trauma-related conditions such as reactive attachment disorder, dissociative disorders or borderline personality disorder, may be exhibiting severe sequelae of early and/or severe childhood trauma, perhaps complicated by other vulnerabilities or risk factors. No controlled treatment studies have specifically addressed the needs of such children. Thus, the traumatized children suffering the greatest functional impairments have received the least attention from treatment researchers. (It is an unfortunate and disturbing corollary that the most symptomatic children, who typically need the most intensive interventions such as wrap around, in home, and residential treatments, usually receive such treatment from the most poorly paid, least trained and least experienced treatment providers.)

## RECOMMENDATIONS FOR FUTURE CLINICAL PRACTICE, RESEARCH AND POLICY

The above summary suggests specific directions for clinical practice, research and policy, which may lead to improved treatment for traumatized children.

### Clinical Practice

Early screening and identification of traumatized children in school, pediatric and other routine settings, and subsequent referral to appropriate treatment will likely improve outcomes for many of these children. Improved efforts to educate pediatric and educational providers about the serious mental health consequences of childhood trauma and PTSD are necessary. Pediatric, mental health and substance abuse treatment providers may also benefit from more specific and intensive training with regard to how to identify traumatized children during clinical assessments, how to provide TF-CBT and other empirically proven treatments if and when they become available, and when and where to refer children who are not responding to such treatments in community treatment settings. As more evidence-based information about the efficacy of pharmacologic treatments is developed, specific algorithms regarding their use should be developed and disseminated to pediatric and psychiatric treatment providers.

### Research

More research is needed to identify effective treatments for traumatized children, including those exposed to a variety of different traumatic events, those with comorbid psychiatric conditions including substance use disorders, and those with serious functional impairments in a variety of domains. Research is also needed regarding the critical components and dosage of TF-CBT, the efficacy of alternative promising treatment models including those provided in the acute aftermath of mass disasters, and the efficacy of psychopharmacological agents used alone or in combination with psychosocial treatments. Multi-site studies employing rigorous scientific methodology are complex and expensive; adequate resources should be allocated in support of such studies, as they are the ones most likely to advance our knowledge about efficacious treatments. In addition to efficacy research, studies regarding how to best transport evidence-based treatments into routine community settings are also needed. The SAMHSA-funded National Child Traumatic Stress Network has established collaborations to empirically examine optimal methods of dissemination, implementation, adoption and adaptation of evidence-based treatments for traumatized children to community treatment providers (www.nctsnet.org). Basic psychobiological research has contributed greatly to our understanding of the physiological mechanisms contributing to the development and maintenance of childhood PTSD (DeBellis et al., 1999). Incorporating psychobiological measures into treatment trials may provide critical information about how to reverse such abnormalities early in the course of this disorder.

## Policy

Clinical practice and research priorities require the availability of adequate funding for child trauma research, including the possibility of dedicating resources specifically to this area. The National Institute of Mental Health has recently earmarked funds for Career Development Awards for child abuse researchers, and the Substance Abuse and Mental Health Services Administration (SAMHSA) has funded the National Child Traumatic Stress Network to encourage high quality child trauma research and treatment. These initiatives have already significantly increased treatment and services development and dissemination for traumatized children; continued funding will no doubt greatly contribute to improved treatment for these children. Maintaining separate funding streams for treating substance use disorders versus other mental health disorders may be a significant barrier to providing optimal services to youth with coexisting PTSD and substance abuse. Better integration of these services is needed to optimally treat such youth (Cohen et al., 2003). Screening children for trauma exposure and PTSD symptomatology in routine settings has policy implications (e.g., legal implications for school personnel who identify reportable child abuse), which need to be considered before such screening is likely to occur. Appropriate policies and financial resources should be developed to facilitate such screening, as early identification and treatment may prevent serious and long-lasting negative sequelae of childhood traumatization. Since psychotherapy has more efficacy evidence than pharmacotherapy for these children, policies should encourage referral to mental health providers rather than favoring the provision of medication in pediatric primary care settings. Given the convincing evidence that including a parental treatment component enhances outcomes for children traumatized by interpersonal violence, insurance coverage for conjoint child and parent treatment should be provided. As more information about optimal treatments for traumatized children becomes available, policy and resource allocation should be adjusted accordingly.

## CONCLUSION

In the wake of the September 11th terrorist attack on the United States, there is growing public awareness of the impact that traumatic exposure has on children and adolescents, and the importance of addressing trauma-related symptoms in a timely manner. Although there have been many recent advances in our knowledge in this regard, changes in clinical practice, research and policy are needed in order to optimally treat traumatized children.

## REFERENCES

Birmaher, B., Ryan, N.D., Brent, D.A., Williamson, D.E., & Kaufman, J. (1996). Child and adolescent depression: A review of the last 10 years. Part II. *Journal of the American Academy of Child and Adolescent Psychiatry, 35,* 1575-1583.

Bisson, J.I., McFarlane, A.C., & Rose, S. (2000). Psychological debriefing. In E.B. Foa, T.M. Keane, & M.J. Friedman (Eds.), *Effective treatments for PTSD: Practice guidelines from the International Society for Traumatic Stress Studies* (pp. 39-59). New York: Guilford Press.

Chaffin, M., Silovsky, J.F., Funderburk, B., Valle, L.A., Brestan, E.V., Balachova, T., Jackson, S., Lensgraf, J., & Bonner, B.L. (2004). Parent-child interaction therapy with physically abusive parents: Efficacy for reducing future abuse reports. *Journal of Consulting and Clinical Psychology, 72,* 500-510.

Chemtob, C.M., Nakashima, J., & Carlson, J.G. (2002). Brief treatment for elementary school children with disaster-related PTSD: A field study. *Journal of Clinical Psychology, 58,* 99-112.

Chemtob, C.M., Nakashima, J.P., & Hamada, R.S. (2002). Psychosocial intervention for postdisaster trauma symptoms in elementary school children. *Archives of Pediatric & Adolescent Medicine, 156*, 211-216.

Cohen, J.A., Berliner, L., & March, J.S. (2000). Treatment of children and adolescents. In E.B. Foa, T.M. Keane, & M.J. Friedman (Eds.), *Effective treatments for PTSD: Practice guidelines from the International Society for Traumatic Stress Studies* (pp. 106-138). New York: Guilford Press.

Cohen, J.A., Deblinger, E., Mannarino, A.P. & Steer, R. (2004). A multisite randomized controlled trial for children with sexual abuse-related PTSD symptoms. *Journal of the American Academy of Child & Adolescent Psychiatry, 43*, 393-402.

Cohen, J.A., Mannarino, A.P., & Knudsen, K. (2005). Treating sexually abused children: One year follow-up of a randomized controlled trial. *Child Abuse & Neglect, 29*, 135-145.

Cohen, J.A., Mannarino, A.P., Zhitova, A.C., & Capone, M. (2003). Treating child abuse-related posttraumatic stress and comorbid substance abuse in adolescents. *Child Abuse & Neglect, 27*, 1345-1365.

Cohen, J.A., Mannarino, A.P., & Rogal, S.S. (2001). Treatment practices for childhood PTSD. *Child Abuse & Neglect, 25*, 123-136.

Cohen, J.A., & Mannarino, A.P. (2000). Predictors of treatment outcome in sexually abused children. *Child Abuse & Neglect, 24*, 983-994.

DeBellis, M.D., Keshavan, M.S., Clark, D.B., Casey, B.J., Giedd, J.N., & Boring, A.M. (1999). Developmental traumatology. Part II: Brain development. *Biological Psychiatry, 45*, 1271-1284.

Deblinger, E., Lippman, J., & Steer, R. (1996). Sexually abused children suffering posttraumatic stress symptoms: Initial treatment outcome findings. *Child Maltreatment, 1*, 310-321.

Field, T., Seligman, S., Scafedi, F., & Schanberg, S. (1996). Alleviating posttraumatic stress in children following Hurricane Andrew. *Journal of Applied Developmental Psychology, 1*:17:37-50.

Foa, E.B., Davidson, J.R.T., & Frances, A. (1999). The expert consensus guideline series: Treatment of PTSD. *Journal of Clinical Psychiatry, 60*(Supplement), 16.

Jaberghaderi, N., Greenwald, R., Rubin, A., Dolatabadim, S., & Zand, S.O. (2002). A comparison of CBT and EMDR for sexually abused Iranian girls. Unpublished manuscript, Allame Tabatabee University, Tehran, Iran.

Kataoka, S.H., Stein, B.D., Jaycox, L.H., Wong, M., Escudero, P., Tu, W., Zaragoza, C., & Fink, A. (2003). A school-based mental health program for traumatized Latino immigrant children. *Journal of the American Academy of Child and Adolescent Psychiatry, 42*, 311-318.

King, N.J., Tonge, B.J., Mullen, P., Myerson, N., Keyne, D., Rollings, S., Martin, R. & Ollendick, T.H. (2000). Treating sexually abused children with posttraumatic stress symptoms: A randomized controlled trial. *Journal of the American Academy of Child and Adolescent Psychiatry, 39*, 1347-1355.

Kolko, D.J. (1996). Individual cognitive behavioral treatment and family therapy for physically abused children and their offending parents: A comparison of clinical outcomes. *Child Maltreatment, 1*, 322-342.

Layne, C.M., Pynoos, S., Saltzman, W.R., Arslanagic, B., Black, M., Savjak, N., Popovic, T., Duakovic, E., Musie, M., Campara, N., Djapo, N., & Houston, R. (2001). Trauma/grief-focused group psychotherapy: School-based postwar intervention with traumatized Bosnian adolescents. *Group Dynamics: Theory, Research & Practice, 5*, 277-290.

March, J., Amaya-Jackson, L., Murray, M., & Schulte, A. (1998). Cognitive-behavioral psychotherapy for children and adolescents with PTSD following a single incident stressor. *Journal of the American Academy of Child and Adolescent Psychiatry, 37*, 585-593.

Perez, C.L. (1998). A comparison of group play therapy and individual therapy for sexually abused children. *Dissertation Abstracts International, 48*, 3079.

Robert, R., Blakeney, P.E., Villarreal, C., Rosenberg, L., & Meyer, W.J. (1999). Imipramine treatment in pediatric burn patients with symptoms of Acute Stress Disorder: A pilot study. *Journal of the American Academy of Child and Adolescent Psychiatry, 38*, 873-882.

Silverman, A.B., Reinherz, H.Z., & Giaconia, R.M. (1996). The long-term sequelae of child and adolescent abuse: A longitudinal community study. *Child Abuse & Neglect, 20*, 709-724.

Stein, B.D., Jaycox, L.H., Kataoka, S.H., Wong, M., Tu, W., Elliott, M.N., & Fink, A. (2003). A mental health intervention for school children exposed to violence: A randomized controlled trial. *Journal of the American Medical Association, 290*, 603-611.

Trowell, J., Kolvin, I., Weeramanthri, T., Sadowski, H., Berelowitz, M., Glasser, D., & Leitch, I. (2002). Psychotherapy for sexually abused girls: Psychopathological outcome findings and patterns of change. *British Journal of Psychiatry, 160*, 234-247.

Trupin, E., Tarico, V., & Low, B. (1993). Children on child protective caseloads: Prevalence and nature of serious emotional disturbance. *Child Abuse & Neglect, 17*, 345-355.

Warshaw, M.G., Fierman, E., Pratt, L., Hunt, M., Yonkers, K.A., Massion, A.O., & Keller, M.B. (1993). Quality of life and dissociation in anxiety disorder patients with history of trauma or PTSD. *American Journal of Psychiatry, 150*, 1512-1516.

# Risk Factor Effect Sizes in PTSD: What This Means for Intervention

## Chris R. Brewin, PhD

**SUMMARY.** This paper reviews evidence concerning the major risk factors for posttraumatic stress disorder. Although there are a number of consistent risk factors, their effects tend to be small and to vary according to the nature of the study. This suggests that they are not well suited to identifying individuals who require early intervention following a traumatic event. In contrast, methods based on symptom reports offer a much more sensitive and practicable approach to screening. A recent instrument, the Trauma Screening Questionnaire, is brief, simple to administer, and highly efficient at identifying survivors in need of intervention. *[Article copies available for a fee from The Haworth Document Delivery Service: 1-800-HAWORTH. E-mail address: <docdelivery@haworthpress.com> Website: <http://www.HaworthPress.com> © 2005 by The Haworth Press, Inc. All rights reserved.]*

**KEYWORDS.** Posttraumatic stress disorder, PTSD, assessment, intervention

Current knowledge about risk factors for posttraumatic stress disorder (PTSD) has important implications for screening and early interven-

---

Chris R. Brewin is Professor of Clinical Psychology, Sub-Department of Clinical Health Psychology, University College London.

Address correspondence to: Chris R. Brewin, PhD, Sub-Department of Clinical Health Psychology, University College London, Gower Street, London WC1E 6BT, UK (E-mail: c.brewin@ucl.ac.uk).

[Haworth co-indexing entry note]: "Risk Factor Effect Sizes in PTSD: What This Means for Intervention." Brewin, Chris R. Co-published simultaneously in *Journal of Trauma & Dissociation* (The Haworth Medical Press, an imprint of The Haworth Press, Inc.) Vol. 6, No. 2, 2005, pp. 123-130; and: *Acute Reactions to Trauma and Psychotherapy: A Multidisciplinary and International Perspective* (ed: Etzel Cardeña, and Kristin Croyle) The Haworth Medical Press, an imprint of The Haworth Press, Inc., 2005, pp. 123-130. Single or multiple copies of this article are available for a fee from The Haworth Document Delivery Service [1-800-HAWORTH, 9:00 a.m. - 5:00 p.m. (EST). E-mail address: docdelivery@haworthpress.com].

doi:10.1300/J229v06n02_11

tion in the management of acute stress. This paper addresses three interrelated questions. First, are risk factors for acute stress disorder (ASD)–which occurs in the first month post-trauma–the same as those for PTSD–a condition that can only be diagnosed after one month post-trauma, but that may become chronic and long-lasting? Second, what do the last 20 years of research on PTSD reveal tell us about the most important risk factors for PTSD and the size of their effects? Third, given what is known about risk factors, what is the most practicable approach to screening individuals for the likelihood that they are suffering from PTSD?

## *ACUTE STRESS DISORDER*
## *AND POSTTRAUMATIC STRESS DISORDER*

Although there has been little research on specific risk factors for ASD, my colleagues and I recently reanalyzed data on acute symptoms experienced by victims of crime within one month post-trauma. By grouping symptoms according to the varying criteria for PTSD and ASD described in the *DSM-IV*, we were able to ascertain the degree of overlap between the two diagnoses (only ignoring the requirement for PTSD symptoms to have been present for more than a month). The analysis revealed a 96% diagnostic overlap between the two conditions, suggesting that they are so similar in nature as to make it extremely likely they share the same risk factors (Brewin, Andrews, & Rose, 2003).

## *RISK FACTORS FOR POSTTRAUMATIC STRESS DISORDER*

A recent meta-analysis summarized current knowledge about risk factors (Brewin, Andrews, & Valentine, 2000). In order to base our conclusions on a homogeneous set of studies we selected articles that fit specific predetermined criteria: they had to be conducted on populations who had all been exposed to a traumatic event in adulthood; the populations had to contain non-disordered as well as disordered participants (thus excluding studies of PTSD in military veterans who all had substance use disorders, for example); each risk factor had to be studied in at least four separate articles; and PTSD had to be measured according to DSM criteria. Using these criteria we identified 14 risk factors (see Table 1).

TABLE 1. Risk Factors for Posttraumatic Stress Disorder (adapted from Brewin, Andrews, & Valentine, 2000)

| | No. of studies | Population size | Weighted average *r* |
|---|---|---|---|
| Risk factors that predict PTSD in some populations only: | | | |
| Female gender | 25 | 11,261 | .13 |
| Younger age | 29 | 7,207 | .06 |
| Race (minority status) | 22 | 8,165 | .05 |
| Risk factors that consistently predict PTSD but to varying extents: | | | |
| Low SES | 18 | 5,957 | .14 |
| Lack of education | 29 | 11,047 | .10 |
| Low intelligence | 6 | 1,149 | .18 |
| Other previous trauma | 14 | 5,147 | .12 |
| Other adverse childhood factors | 14 | 6,969 | .19 |
| Trauma severity | 49 | 13,653 | .23 |
| Lack of social support | 11 | 3,276 | .40 |
| Life stress | 8 | 2,804 | .32 |
| Risk factors with homogeneous effects in predicting PTSD: | | | |
| Psychiatric history | 22 | 7,307 | .11 |
| Childhood abuse | 9 | 1,746 | .14 |
| Family psychiatric history | 11 | 4,792 | .13 |

Meta-analysis does not allow the investigator to examine relationships between variables within a study, only across studies. Therefore we were unable to look at the interaction between individual risk factors and were obliged to conduct separate meta-analyses on each one. We were, however, able to examine the effect of important study parameters that might influence the impact of each risk factor; these included the type of trauma (military versus civilian), the gender of participants, whether the study used a retrospective or a prospective design, whether PTSD was measured by the presence or absence of a diagnosis or by continuous symptom scores, whether PTSD was measured by interview or questionnaire, and whether the sample included some participants whose traumas might have occurred in childhood. This last factor was necessary so that we could include ten large and influential epidemiological studies, which were a source of valuable information.

By searching databases such as PILOTS (a specialist resource maintained by the National Center for PTSD), hand-searching relevant

journals, inspecting reference lists in journal articles, and contacting individual researchers, we eventually located 85 datasets derived from 77
separate articles. The sample sizes ranged from 25 to 4,127. The majority of the articles (49) were based on civilian samples, compared to 28
articles concerning military populations. Most of the articles (59) were
purely retrospective but 18 were at least partly longitudinal, i.e., risk
factor data were collected either prior to the trauma or post-trauma but
prior to the development of PTSD. All but 4 studies measured PTSD using *DSM-III* or *DSM-IIIR* criteria.

Table 1 shows the number of studies, the total sample size, and the
average effect size *r* for each risk factor. This statistic can vary between
0 and 1, with larger *r* denoting a stronger risk. Values of *r* are weighted
according to sample size, so that larger studies contribute more to the
overall estimate. On the basis of our analysis it is convenient to divide
the risk factors into three groups. The first group consists of factors that
were associated with increased risk in some types of study but not at all
in others. The overall impact of two of these factors, younger age and
race (minority status), was very small, and their effects were only apparent in military settings. In contrast, female gender was only a risk factor
in civilian settings.

The second group of risk factors consists of those that consistently
predicted PTSD in all studies but to significantly varying extents. Like
the first group, therefore, their role was more important in some types of
study than in others. For example, lack of education, general childhood
adversity, trauma severity, and lack of social support were more important in military than in civilian studies. In general, pre-trauma risk
factors had lower average effect sizes than trauma severity or the post-
trauma factors of additional life stress and social support. However, this
may be partly because there was less scope for their estimates to be inflated by the effect of existing PTSD. Retrospective reports of trauma
severity, support, etc., may have been magnified by response biases in
participants who had already developed PTSD.

The third group of risk factors, consisting of the presence of a previous psychiatric history, a family psychiatric history, or reported abuse
in childhood, were the most reliable in the sense that their effects were
moderate in size and did not vary systematically across different types
of study.

As can be seen, the effect of most of the fourteen risk factors varied
according to at least some of the different study parameters. Three were
impacted by the gender of participants, three by whether the design was
retrospective or prospective, six by whether investigators used a diag-

nosis or continuous scores, four by the use of an interview versus a questionnaire, and six by whether participants with childhood traumas were included. In particular, the risk associated with gender, age, and trauma severity varied considerably, being affected by five out of the six study parameters investigated. In conclusion, the meta-analysis demonstrated a number of important things. First, most risk factors had small to moderate effects that varied according to the type of study being conducted. PTSD in military samples had a markedly different profile of risk factors than did PTSD in civilian samples. Trauma severity and post-trauma risk factors appeared to be more important than pre-trauma factors, but their measurement was vulnerable to retrospective bias.

Another recent meta-analysis (Ozer, Best, Lipsey, & Weiss, 2003) replicated some of the above findings and identified additional risk factors occurring during the trauma itself. Perceived threat to life, intense peri-traumatic emotions, and greater peri-traumatic dissociation (depersonalization, derealization, out-of-body experiences, etc.) were all associated with a greater risk of subsequent PTSD. Effect sizes were moderate, ranging from .26 for threat to life and emotional reactions to .35 for dissociation, and are likely to be somewhat inflated by retrospective bias. Whereas dissociative reactions that specifically occur during or in the immediate aftermath of the trauma are consistently related to later PTSD, the occurrence of similar reactions in the days and weeks after the trauma is over does not always have the same predictive value (e.g., Brewin, Andrews, Rose, & Kirk, 1999).

## SCREENING FOR POSTTRAUMATIC STRESS DISORDER

Given the limited predictive power of the most prominent risk factors, how can those survivors of traumatic events likely to develop PTSD or already suffering from PTSD be efficiently identified? The alternative approach has been to rely on the presence of early symptoms of reexperiencing, avoidance and numbing, and arousal taken from the *DSM-IV* (American Psychiatric Association, 2000). Providing these symptoms are not measured too soon post-trauma, consistent and relatively strong predictive effects have been obtained. Most existing instruments involve the use of rating scales and decision rules, and contain 17 items or more (see Brewin et al., 2003, for a review). Recently studies have investigated the performance of 4-, 6-, and 12-item screening instruments requiring respondents to rate the frequency and/

or severity of subsets of these symptoms. These have shown promising results equivalent to longer 17-item measures, although none have yet been validated on independent samples.

Our own studies have shown (Brewin et al., 1999) that victims of violent crime at high risk of developing PTSD six months later could be identified by their reports at three weeks post-crime of at least three reexperiencing or at least three arousal symptoms, all present at moderate intensity. Although previous studies have suggested that the avoidance and numbing symptom cluster may be most efficient for screening purposes, because it is less common to reach the threshold for these symptoms than it is for the reexperiencing and arousal symptoms (e.g., North et al., 1999), this is probably due to the fact that more symptoms are required to meet the criterion. If equivalent numbers of reexperiencing or arousal symptoms are required, our data indicated that prediction is just as good. These findings suggested that the identification of individuals currently suffering from PTSD or at risk of developing PTSD could be made much simpler than current methods allow. In a subsequent study we therefore developed a brief 10-item screening instrument based solely on *DSM-IV* reexperiencing and arousal symptoms. Simplicity was obtained by omitting avoidance and numbing symptoms, and by requiring a simple Yes or No to the question whether the symptom had been experienced at least twice in the past week.

The new Trauma Screening Questionnaire has been tested on samples of rail crash survivors and cross-validated on victims of violent crime (Brewin et al., 2002). Requiring respondents to endorse at least six out of the ten reexperiencing or arousal symptoms, in any combination, led to high levels of sensitivity (.86, .76) and specificity (.93, .97), with excellent positive (.86, .91) and negative (.93, .92) predictive power. In both samples the overall efficiency of the instrument exceeded 90%. The figures are equivalent to the level of agreement previously obtained between the two most highly regarded interview assessments currently available for PTSD, the Structured Clinical Interview for *DSM-IV* (SCID) PTSD module and the CAPS (Blake et al., 1995). The Trauma Screening Questionnaire has the additional advantage that it is quick and easy to use, requiring no knowledge of PTSD or its diagnostic criteria.

## CONCLUSIONS

The results of the two meta-analyses suggest that it is probably impractical to attempt to identify individuals at risk for PTSD from their pre-trauma characteristics, or from their subjective accounts of trauma severity, peri-traumatic reactions, or later environmental factors. A much more promising approach is to track early symptoms and identify individuals whose symptoms do not improve. The length of time this may take will depend on the severity of the trauma and on complicating factors such as injury and bereavement. However, for the majority of everyday assaults and accidents we can expect symptoms to be in decline by three to four weeks post-trauma. Given the lack of any evidence for the value of brief early interventions such as critical incident stress debriefing (Rose & Bisson, 1998; Rose, Bisson, & Wessely, 2004), an alternative approach, which we have called "Screen and Treat," is indicated. This involves allowing natural recovery processes to run their course with as little interference as possible for the first few weeks, but screening individuals with instruments such as the Trauma Screening Questionnaire to ensure that recovery does indeed take place. In the absence of recovery, empirically validated treatments for PTSD should be offered. It is likely that this form of early intervention will lead to more efficient targeting of resources while at the same time capitalizing on natural recovery processes and reaping the benefit of addressing symptoms before they have become chronic.

## REFERENCES

American Psychiatric Association. (2000). *Diagnostic and statistical manual of mental disorders, 4th ed., text revision.* Washington, DC: Author.

Blake, D.D., Weathers, F.W., Nagy, L.M., Kaloupek, D.G., Gusman, F.D., Charney, D.S., & Keane, T.M. (1995). The development of a clinician-administered PTSD scale. *Journal of Traumatic Stress, 8,* 75-90.

Brewin, C.R., Andrews, B., & Rose, S. (2003). Diagnostic overlap between acute stress disorder and posttraumatic stress disorder in victims of violent crime. *American Journal of Psychiatry, 160,* 783-785.

Brewin, C.R., Andrews, B., Rose, S., & Kirk, M. (1999). Acute stress disorder and posttraumatic stress disorder in victims of violent crime. *American Journal of Psychiatry, 156,* 360-366.

Brewin, C.R., Andrews, B., & Valentine, J.D. (2000). Meta-analysis of risk factors for posttraumatic stress disorder in trauma-exposed adults. *Journal of Consulting and Clinical Psychology, 68,* 748-766.

Brewin, C.R., Rose, S., & Andrews, B. (2003). Screening for posttraumatic stress disorder in civilian populations. In R. Ørner & U. Schnyder (Eds.), *Reconstructing early intervention after trauma* (pp. 130-142). Oxford: Oxford University Press.

Brewin, C.R., Rose, S., Andrews, B., Green, J., Tata, P., McEvedy, C., Turner, S.W., & Foa, E.B. (2002). A brief screening instrument for posttraumatic stress disorder. *British Journal of Psychiatry, 181,* 158-162.

North, C.S., Nixon, S.J., Shariat, S., Mallonee, S., McMillen, J.C., Spitznagel, E.L., & Smith, E.M. (1999). Psychiatric disorders among survivors of the Oklahoma City bombing. *Journal of the American Medical Association, 282*, 755-762.

Ozer, E.J., Best, S.R., Lipsey, T.L., & Weiss, D.S. (2003). Predictors of posttraumatic stress disorder and symptoms in adults: A meta-analysis. *Psychological Bulletin, 129*, 52-73.

Rose, S., & Bisson, J.I. (1998). Brief early psychological interventions following trauma: A systematic review of the literature. *Journal of Traumatic Stress, 11*, 697-710.

Rose, S., Bisson, J., & Wessely, S. (2004). Psychological debriefing for preventing post-traumatic stress disorder (PTSD) (Cochrane Review). In *The Cochrane Library* (Issue 3). Chichester, UK: John Wiley & Sons, Ltd.

# Index

# BOOK ORDER FORM!

Order a copy of this book with this form or online at:
http://www.HaworthPress.com/store/product.asp?sku=5645

## Acute Reactions to Trauma and Psychotherapy
### *A Multidisciplinary and International Perspective*

____ in softbound at $19.95 ISBN-13: 978-0-7890-2974-4 / ISBN-10: 0-7890-2974-X.
____ in hardbound at $34.95 ISBN-13: 978-0-7890-2973-7 / ISBN-10: 0-7890-2973-1.

COST OF BOOKS _____

POSTAGE & HANDLING _____
US: $4.00 for first book & $1.50
for each additional book
Outside US: $5.00 for first book
& $2.00 for each additional book.

SUBTOTAL _____

In Canada: add 7% GST. _____

STATE TAX _____
CA, IL, IN, MN, NJ, NY, OH, PA & SD residents
please add appropriate local sales tax.

FINAL TOTAL _____
If paying in Canadian funds, convert
using the current exchange rate,
UNESCO coupons welcome.

❑BILL ME LATER:
Bill-me option is good on US/Canada/
Mexico orders only; not good to jobbers,
wholesalers, or subscription agencies.

❑Signature _____

❑Payment Enclosed: $ _____

❑ PLEASE CHARGE TO MY CREDIT CARD:
❑Visa ❑MasterCard ❑AmEx ❑Discover
❑Diner's Club ❑Eurocard ❑ JCB

Account #_____

Exp Date _____

Signature _____
*(Prices in US dollars and subject to change without notice.)*

| PLEASE PRINT ALL INFORMATION OR ATTACH YOUR BUSINESS CARD |
|---|

Name

Address

City          State/Province          Zip/Postal Code

Country

Tel          Fax

E-Mail

May we use your e-mail address for confirmations and other types of information? ❑Yes ❑No We appreciate receiving
your e-mail address. Haworth would like to e-mail special discount offers to you, as a preferred customer.
**We will never share, rent, or exchange your e-mail address.** We regard such actions as an invasion of your privacy.

Order from your **local bookstore** or directly from
**The Haworth Press, Inc.** 10 Alice Street, Binghamton, New York 13904-1580 • USA
Call our toll-free number (1-800-429-6784) / Outside US/Canada: (607) 722-5857
Fax: 1-800-895-0582 / Outside US/Canada: (607) 771-0012
E-mail your order to us: orders@HaworthPress.com

**For orders outside US and Canada,** you may wish to order through your local
sales representative, distributor, or bookseller.
For information, see http://HaworthPress.com/distributors

*(Discounts are available for individual orders in US and Canada only, not booksellers/distributors.)*

The
Haworth
Press
Inc.

**Please photocopy this form for your personal use.**
www.HaworthPress.com

BOF05